THE EVERYTHING

FERTILITY

BOOK

Dear Reader,

While conceiving a baby can certainly happen unexpectedly, it quite often requires a great deal of planning and preparation. The decision to have a baby is often one that brings great joy and happiness to everyone surrounding the couple.

Every year, however, thousands of couples face the heartache and confusion that accompanies the moment they recognize that this may not be the easy, natural process they envisioned. Unless you know someone who has struggled with infertility, you may be filled with fear and anxiety when beginning treatment. Is there something wrong with me? With my partner? Will we ever have children?

As an infertility nurse, I've worked with hundreds of couples in the same situation as you. I've shared their joys, their sorrows, and the uncertainty in between.

I hope this book gives you the information you need to make informed decisions about your care. I hope the little tips I've shared make the process just a bit easier for you. And most of all, I hope that the end of this journey brings you the little bundle of joy you have been wishing for.

Best of luck!

Nicole Galan, RN

Welcome to the EVERYTHING® Series!

These handy, accessible books give you all you need to tackle a difficult project, gain a new hobby, comprehend a fascinating topic, prepare for an exam, or even brush up on something you learned back in school but have since forgotten.

You can choose to read an *Everything*® book from cover to cover or just pick out the information you want from our four useful boxes: e-questions, e-facts, e-alerts, and e-ssentials.

We give you everything you need to know on the subject, but throw in a lot of fun stuff along the way, too.

We now have more than 400 *Everything*® books in print, spanning such wide-ranging categories as weddings, pregnancy, cooking, music instruction, foreign language, crafts, pets, New Age, and so much more. When you're done reading them all, you can finally say you know *Everything*®!

QUESTION

Answers to common questions

FACT

Important snippets of information

ALERT

Urgent warnings

ESSENTIAL

Quick handy tips

PUBLISHER Karen Cooper

DIRECTOR OF ACQUISITIONS AND INNOVATION Paula Munier

MANAGING EDITOR, EVERYTHING® SERIES Lisa Laing

COPY CHIEF Casey Ebert

ASSISTANT PRODUCTION EDITOR Jacob Erickson

ACQUISITIONS EDITOR Katrina Schroeder

ASSOCIATE DEVELOPMENT EDITOR Hillary Thompson

EDITORIAL ASSISTANT Ross Weisman

EVERYTHING® SERIES COVER DESIGNER Erin Alexander

LAYOUT DESIGNERS Colleen Cunningham, Elisabeth Lariviere, Ashley Vierra, Denise Wallace

Visit the entire Everything® series at *www.everything.com*

THE
EVERYTHING®
FERTILITY
BOOK

All you need to know about fertility, conception,
and a healthy pregnancy

Nicole Galan, RN

Foreword by Richard V. Grazi, MD

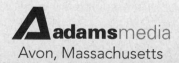

Adamsmedia
Avon, Massachusetts

To my Tommy:
thank you for always pushing and
encouraging me to work toward my dreams.

An Everything® Series Book.
Everything® and everything.com® are registered trademarks of F+W Media, Inc.

Published by Adams Media, a division of F+W Media, Inc.
57 Littlefield Street, Avon, MA 02322 U.S.A.
www.adamsmedia.com

Contains material adapted and abridged from *The Everything® Getting Pregnant Book*
by Robin Elise Weiss, copyright © 2004 by F+W Media, Inc.,
ISBN 10: 1-59337-034-2, ISBN 13: 978-1-59337-034-3.

ISBN 10: 1-4405-0546-2
ISBN 13: 978-1-4405-0546-1
eISBN 10: 1-4405-0547-0
eISBN 13: 978-1-4405-0547-8

Printed in the United States of America.

10 9 8 7 6 5 4 3 2 1

Library of Congress Cataloging-in-Publication Data
Galan, Nicole.
The everything fertility book / Nicole Galan.
p. cm.
Includes bibliographical references and index.
ISBN 978-1-4405-0546-1 (alk. paper)
1. Infertility—Popular works. 2. Fertility, Human—Popular works. 3. Conception. I. Title.
RC889.G28   2011
616.6'92—dc22   2010039120

This book is available at quantity discounts for bulk purchases.
For information, please call 1-800-289-0963.

Contents

Acknowledgments

The journey infertility forces some to take is infinitely personal and private. Therefore, I must thank the countless patients who have shared their struggles with me on a daily basis.

To the incredible staff I work with—I have never seen such a dedicated group of professionals who care so deeply about their patients. Without the work that you do, thousands of families would be incomplete.

Dr. Grazi and Dr. Seifer—thank you for sharing your depth of knowledge with me. The autonomy, respect, and recognition you provide your employees in general and your nurses in particular is second to none.

To the nursing staff, and especially Joanne, Natalya, Erica, Toby W., and Rosa—thank you, thank you, thank you for teaching me everything you know about infertility. I could not have learned as much as I have without your endless knowledge, patience, and unique ability to truly advocate for your patients.

My mom and dad—thank you for being amazing parents and teaching me how to reach for my dreams. Thank you also for teaching me how to be an incredible mom. I love you both so much.

For my sister Jenn, who is always there to listen and be my partner in crime, be it with pints of ice cream or trips to the spa.

For Carmela; you make me proud to be a nurse.

Thank you to my entire family, and Maria in particular, for the extra babysitting hours you've put in. I could not have done this without your support.

For Jackson, my own little miracle. I am so eternally grateful and blessed to be your mamacita. I love you in a way that I didn't know was possible until I met you.

And finally, for Tommy. You've stood with me when I needed help and pushed me to walk by myself when I needed to find my own strength. You've been my partner, my support, and my coach. Your endless perseverance has been a source of inspiration to me and I am so incredibly lucky to be sharing this journey of life with you. Thank you a thousand times over. I love you.

The Top 10 Things
You Need to Know Before
Beginning Fertility Treatment

1. You are not alone. Thousands of couples go through this every year.

2. Choose the clinic you go to very carefully.

3. Never hesitate to get a second opinion.

4. Do anything you can to help reduce your stress—get regular massages, try acupuncture, or make extra time for yourself during the day.

5. Keep working on your marriage and intimate life. Fertility treatment can be a real drain on spontaneity and intimacy.

6. Keep your weight at a healthy level.

7. Make sure to take a prenatal vitamin every day and eat plenty of fruits and vegetables to ensure that you are getting all of the nutrients you need.

8. Get extra support if you need it. This includes individual and marital counseling if necessary.

9. Stop smoking and drinking and be more mindful of your caffeine intake.

10. Read up on the workings of your body. Possessing a basic understanding can help you have a more meaningful discussion with your doctor.

Foreword

Most of us grow up expecting that, like our parents before us, we will have children at some point in our lives. We embark on starting a family without entertaining the possibility that our plan may fail. When a couple discovers that their efforts do not result in a pregnancy, their situation is often accompanied by shock, confusion, and fear. Infertility is more than just a medical condition; it is a crisis that can affect every aspect of a couple's life together. Fortunately, there are solutions that can help most couples achieve a healthy pregnancy and birth. But, as so many women and men already know, overcoming infertility is not always easy.

The Everything® Fertility Book is an essential companion to those who must navigate the pathway from infertility to parenthood. Drawing from her years of experience as a nurse working in the field of assisted reproduction, Nicole Galan, RN, has compiled a treasure trove of information that will help those in need make their way successfully through diagnosis and treatment. Her presentation is clear, concise, and demystifies the entire process for those who are unfamiliar with the modern medical management of infertility.

It is with great pride that I accepted Nicole's request to review her manuscript. What was evident as I read through it was how well she was able to distill the practical, day-to-day issues that our patients face, and then lay them out in a way that beginning patients can understand and digest, as well as those who have been trying to conceive over a longer period of time. Our years of working together at Genesis have clearly borne fruit.

Of course, this book is not meant to replace appropriate professional care. Still, it is a very good place to start. In sharing her detailed understanding of infertility and its management, Nicole has made sure to explore the challenges faced not only by traditional couples, but also by single women and same-sex couples. In addition, she includes discussion of alternative medicine, a commonly pursued approach by many patients.

The importance of a book like this cannot be overstated. Those of us who work with infertile couples and individuals know how daunting it is to be a patient, especially when the most intimate aspects of life become subject to scrutiny and manipulation. Most patients find that the more detailed their understanding is of the problems they face, the more empowered they feel in making decisions about their care. With *The Everything® Fertility Book* as a resource, those struggling with infertility will better understand the language of their caregivers and the rationale behind their approach. Ultimately, this will make them more involved—and more comfortable—in accessing the care they need. As many have already discovered, becoming an active participate in this process is often the key to success.

—RICHARD V. GRAZI, MD
Founder and Director
Genesis Fertility and Reproductive Medicine

Introduction

IT GOES WITHOUT SAYING that infertility can be a heartbreaking issue for the thousands of couples it affects each year. What seems like such a natural process can quickly turn into a nightmarish process of testing, medications, ultrasounds, injections, and sometimes even surgery. For the couple going through it, the process is confusing, scary, and incredibly unfair. Having a good doctor and fertility clinic to help you medically is only the beginning.

You must also be thoroughly equipped for everything that this process has to offer. You should find simple things you can do at home to boost your own fertility before getting to the clinic, find alternative methods that can help you relax, and establish a strong support system you can lean on during times of stress and challenge. All of these elements are absolutely essential to successfully navigating the world of infertility treatment.

Without having the essential information, an already difficult process can be made even more so. Understanding what is about to happen can help you both take control over your fertility and use the vast amount of information out there to find something that works for you. There are a number of ways that you can help boost your own inherent fertility—diet, herbal supplements, yoga, and acupuncture have all been reported as methods that will help your body conceive a pregnancy.

There are also a good number of techniques you can use at home, before consulting with a specialist. Did you know that your body temperature can be a powerful tool in helping you detect your most fertile time? Or that a simple urine dipstick available at most pharmacies can help you better time when you should have intercourse to conceive? These simple techniques can help you avoid seeing a doctor all together.

As technology is evolving and couples are talking about their struggles more, there has been an explosion of information and resources available both on the Internet and through your doctor's office. Chances are good you even know somebody who is going through the very same thing.

It is vital that you use the available information to help guide your treatment. You are not at the mercy of your physician; getting the information for yourself and advocating for your care is essential. It also helps you work with your doctor in a productive manner to get you to your ultimate goal—a child.

Use the information in this book to help you navigate this unfamiliar terrain. Have an understanding of what is out there, what your options are, and what you feel comfortable with, and know that not every treatment protocol is right for everyone. This field is ripe with ethical debates—genetic screening, egg donation, international surrogacy—and the topics that are encompassed in reproductive technology would make an ethicist's head spin. That being said, you should only do what is right for you and your family.

The good news is that most couples do end up fulfilling their dream of having a child at some point over the course of their treatment. She may not be their biological child or genetic offspring, but she is still their child, regardless of how she came into their lives. If you find yourselves in the unfortunate position where having your own child is no longer an option, there are a number of resources at the end of this book that can help you determine if adoption or fostering a child is right for you. There is also information about finding satisfaction in living your life without children.

CHAPTER 1

Do We Need
Infertility Treatment?

Getting pregnant seems like it should be a natural process, so it can be unnerving when conception doesn't happen right away. When exactly, couples often wonder, is it appropriate to seek out the advice of a fertility specialist? Before going down that road, there are a few things that you can try at home to boost your own fertility, and this chapter will help you use these techniques. Of course, there are special circumstances that warrant treatment much sooner.

Getting the Timing Right

It's often fun and exciting when couples first start trying to conceive. The process seems simple enough; you only need to have sex in order to become pregnant. In fact, there is only a specific window of opportunity each month when a woman can become pregnant.

Each month at a specific moment in her menstrual cycle, a woman releases an egg from her ovary, a process known as ovulation. When that egg is fertilized with a single sperm cell, the egg and sperm each contribute half of the genetic material for the embryo. If the egg and sperm aren't in the same place at the right time, fertilization and pregnancy cannot occur. There are a number of methods you can use at home to help you more efficiently time when ovulation is occurring, and thus, when to have sex.

Ovulation Predictor Kits

Perhaps the most well-known and widely used method is the ovulation predictor kit. Available over the counter, these sticks detect the level of luteinizing hormone, or LH, in your urine. Your LH levels surge right before ovulation occurs, triggering the positive result on the stick. It is important to read the instructions very carefully, as each brand has its own way of alerting you.

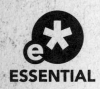

ESSENTIAL

Understanding your own menstrual cycle is absolutely essential when trying to get pregnant. Keep track of your cycles for a month or two to determine how long your cycles are (from the start of one period to the start of the next). Ovulation usually occurs fourteen days before your next menstrual period.

Starting around day ten of your cycle (day one is the first day of full flow bleeding), use one predictor stick every morning, or every other morning, when you first urinate after waking up. A kit showing a positive result means that ovulation is imminent and you can begin having intercourse. When it comes to sex for conception, more isn't necessarily better. Experts agree that having intercourse two to three times around the time of ovulation is optimal. Any more and your partner's sperm count may be affected.

Basal Body Temperature

Your body temperature is very sensitive and is affected by changes in your body's hormonal levels. Measuring the minute changes that occur on a daily basis can give you a clue as to when ovulation is about to occur. There are thermometers available that are specifically marketed as basal body thermometers, but you can use any one that measures temperature to the nearest tenth of a degree. Both digital and glass thermometers work, though digital thermometers are usually quicker and easier to read.

To measure your basal body temperature, simply take your temperature first thing every morning. You will want to take your temperature before you do anything else, including going to the bathroom, speaking, sitting, or standing up. Make sure to leave the thermometer, along with a pen and paper, next to your bedside so that it is readily available when you wake up. This way everything will be ready for you and you can minimize how much you move around in the morning.

You should track your temperature consistently every day from the start of one period to the start of the next. Even seemingly minor changes can throw off the accuracy of your charting. It may even take several cycles before you see a pattern that you can work from.

ALERT

If you use a glass thermometer, remember to shake it down before you go to bed at night. This will prevent you from altering your basal body temperature when you wake up. If you forget and have to shake it down in the morning, your basal body temperature reading will be inaccurate.

During the first part of your cycle, you will have lower temperatures than during the latter part. To identify ovulation, you should look for at least a 0.4 degree rise over your average basal body temperature over the course of a couple of days. You may also notice a slight drop in temperature right before ovulation occurs. The longer you chart, the easier it will be to track your fertile days.

Your peak temperature should be the highest number you recorded over the previous days. Occasionally, an inaccurate temperature will get in your chart for a variety of reasons. This is usually because of a passing illness or mistake being made when you took your temperature; you will learn how to pinpoint these more easily the longer you chart. When a temperature shift occurs and stays high for three consecutive days, you can assume you are ovulating. You have gone from the follicular phase into the next phase of your chart—the luteal phase.

Typically, the luteal phase lasts for the rest of your cycle. If you do not become pregnant, your basal body temperatures will shift back down to the averages found during the follicular phase as you once again begin your menstrual flow. If you become pregnant, your basal body temperatures tend to stay higher, above the temperatures you had earlier in the cycle. This is one way to tell if you are pregnant.

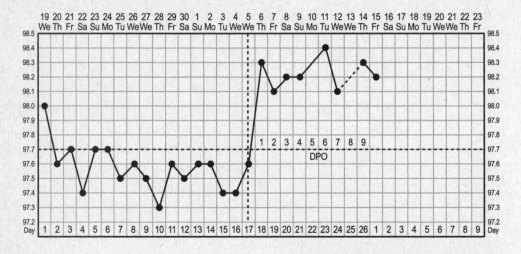

Basal body temperature chart

Checking Your Cervical Mucus

Cervical mucus is a substance that surrounds your cervix and helps to bring the sperm into the uterus after intercourse. It changes in color and consistency as you get closer to ovulation. By examining your cervical mucus on a daily basis, you should begin to notice subtle differences around the midpoint of your cycle.

To begin, wash your hands and under your nails thoroughly as you do not want to introduce bacteria into your vagina. You can get a sample of cervical mucus in one of two ways, the first of which is to use toilet paper to gently wipe the outer opening of your vagina. If you are not able to get an adequate sample that way, you can insert one or two fingers into your vagina and locate your cervix. Find the cervical opening and remove a small amount of mucus. If you are having difficulty locating your cervix, you may need to change position or have your partner help you.

ALERT

Talk to your doctor if you don't notice changes in your cervical mucus after checking it for several months. Poor cervical mucus can affect conception and can sometimes be treated with medication.

Once you've removed a small sample of your mucus, observe the color and consistency, and then stretch it between two fingers. On nonfertile days, your mucus is opaque, thick, and will not stretch well. As ovulation nears, the mucus will thin out and become clear in color. For that reason, fertile mucus is often referred to as being of "egg white consistency." It will stretch to a distance of several inches when you pull your fingers apart. It may take a few months before you can easily distinguish between fertile and nonfertile mucus. However, this change signals an impending ovulation, and you should begin having sex.

Checking the Position of Your Cervix

Another great fertility signal your body offers is the positioning of your cervix. The mouth to your uterus actually moves within your vagina. During the majority of your cycle the cervix is less accessible to sperm. As you get closer to ovulation, the cervix moves. The opening becomes oriented more toward the center of the vagina, where sperm is most likely to be deposited.

Checking your cervix is relatively simple: simply wash your hands and insert your index finger. If you have trouble reaching your cervix, look for alternative positions. Feel for the opening of the cervix in relation to the vagina.

Checking the position of your cervix is not necessarily something that you can do in one day. The idea is to get an impression of when changes are taking place; you will begin to notice this over time. You will also be able to tell when the position is being altered for reasons other than fertility, like when your bowels are full, for example.

There can be different indications that the position of your cervix has changed. Sometimes you or your partner might notice it during sexual intercourse. You may find that the tip of his penis seems to be hitting something; that something is usually your cervix during fertile times. Keep in mind that this contact will not hurt your cervix.

If your partner is checking the position of your cervix, he will notice these changes over time as well. Because of this, it is best to have the same person, be it you or your partner, check the position of the cervix during a given cycle. This will help with consistency and ease of charting.

The Consistency of Your Cervix

The consistency of your cervix means how it feels to the touch. As you begin to feel your cervix more often, you'll notice that the feeling of the tissues changes. These changes are related to the hormones in your cycle; the closer you are to ovulation, the softer the cervical tissues are to the touch.

FACT

The cervical tissues will change from feeling as hard as the tip of your nose to feeling softer, like the lobe of your ear or the inside of your cheek. These adjustments are caused by hormonal changes in your body as it prepares for ovulation and potential pregnancy.

When you feel the tip of your cervix, pay attention to how hard or soft the cervix feels. Again, the cervix becomes softer as you get closer to ovulating. You may also notice that the tip is slightly more open. This is another way your body tries to help you achieve pregnancy.

What Is Secondary Infertility?

Many couples believe that once they've had a baby, having subsequent children will be just as easy. It's often surprising when infertility strikes while trying for a first, second, or even third child. This difficulty conceiving other children is called secondary infertility. It is not considered secondary infertility if your first child was conceived using fertility treatment. Primary infertility occurs when a woman has difficulty conceiving her first child.

What Causes Secondary Infertility?

Just like primary infertility, there are many different factors that can cause secondary infertility. Sometimes the cause is fairly obvious (e.g., if you or your partner has had surgery or an illness which directly affects the reproductive organs). If you've had a previous Cesarean section, the surgery may have caused scarring of the uterine wall that can affect your ability to get pregnant.

It's also very important to remember that your natural fertility declines from year to year as well. Even through you had your first child easily at the age of thirty-three, waiting until the age of thirty-eight before trying for your next child may cause significant problems the second time around. A woman's fertility significantly declines around the age of thirty-five and decreases more so each following year. The rate of genetic diseases and abnormalities also increases dramatically as a woman ages.

Coping with Secondary Infertility

Couples facing secondary infertility have unique needs and issues. They often struggle with feelings of guilt over not being grateful for the children they already have or for not being able to provide them with siblings. Family and friends may even directly ask when the next one is coming along. And yet, given the fact that they have children, it may be uncomfortable connecting with other couples dealing with primary infertility.

What you share with others is entirely up to you. Your family and friends are of course very important to you and you may feel comfortable sharing your struggles to conceive again. Then again, you may not. It can be helpful to have a discussion with your partner about who you plan to tell what. This ensures that you are both on the same page, and nobody is surprised by a distant relative asking very personal questions. If you decide to talk to your family about it, be prepared for questions. Most people have never heard of secondary infertility and are probably not trying to be insensitive.

FACT

There are a number of major organizations that can provide support and information. Check out *www.resolve.org*, *www.inciid.org*, and *www.asrm.org* for more information and for help finding a local or Internet support group. Another great source of information is the nursing staff at your doctor's office. They are often aware of and can direct you to local programs.

Talking to Your Children about Secondary Infertility

One of the most difficult aspects of secondary infertility is talking to your children about it. They may be wondering why they don't have any brothers or sisters and may ask you, quite incessantly, for siblings. And of course, they don't understand that you may be trying and having difficulty.

So what should you tell your child? The answer to that depends on their age, maturity level, and your own comfort level. Some parents choose to tell their children that they are trying to have a baby and need some help from the doctor to do so. Others choose not to tell their children anything at all until they are pregnant and are confident in the pregnancy, particularly if they've had multiple losses. Be aware that children are very observant and have active imaginations. They may become concerned when they see that you are visiting the doctor, and overhear you whispering about the blood tests and treatments that you may frequently require in the coming months. Further, it is just as important to not give your children too much information and displace your own feelings of fear and grief onto them.

Should I Talk to My Gynecologist?

Physicians are now recommending that you see your gynecologist for an appointment dedicated to preconception counseling. The purpose of this appointment is to discuss optimizing your health for pregnancy; topics covered in these meetings include what your weight should be, and whether you need to lose (or gain) prior to becoming pregnant. You'll discuss any foods that you should eat or avoid, what role exercise should play, and what activities are safe and which ones aren't. Finally, it's also a great opportunity to discuss any health issues that may impact your pregnancy.

There are many gynecologists who will treat infertility in the preliminary stages. For example, if you know that you have polycystic ovary syndrome or do not have regular menstrual cycles, these doctors can prescribe a medication called Clomid, which can induce ovulation. However, it is important to know that Clomid often produces several egg follicles (and thus eggs) on the ovaries, putting you at a greater risk of having multiples.

If you are not pregnant within a few cycles, your physician will most likely refer you to a reproductive endocrinologist (RE) for more specialized treatment.

When Should We See an Infertility Specialist?

The golden rule for infertility treatment is that you should be evaluated if you are younger than thirty-five and have been trying unsuccessfully for over a year, or if you are older than thirty-five and have been trying for six months or more.

There are exceptions to this rule, however. Having had multiple miscarriages or pregnancy losses is an indication that you may need help figuring out the cause. If you know that you or your partner has a medical or genetic issue that may impact your fertility, it may be beneficial to see the doctor much earlier. Examples of such medical conditions include:

- Varicoceles (essentially a varicose vein in the penis)
- Certain genetic diseases
- Uterine fibroids
- Endometriosis
- Structural defects in the reproductive organs
- Irregular or absent menstrual cycles
- Polycystic ovary syndrome

All should be evaluated by your gynecologist (or urologist in the case of male factor infertility), who may be able to offer preliminary advice or even recommend that you see a RE immediately.

No Partner, No Problem!

Many single women are opting to have children on their own, before getting married. You may choose this road for a variety of reasons. Maybe you are ready to have children and aren't married, or don't plan on getting married any time soon. You may be concerned about aging and not being able to have children once you are married. Whatever the reason, there are a multitude of options you can pursue.

The Other Half of the Equation

The most obvious issue is where you will get the sperm needed for treatment. Sperm can come from an anonymous donor, usually purchased at a sperm bank, or it can come from someone you know, like a friend or even nonblood-related family member. There are advantages and disadvantages to either option, so deciding on a sperm donor requires a great deal of thought. Most fertility centers offer the services of a reproductive psychologist, a mental health professional with additional training in counseling patients undergoing reproductive therapies. This person can help you weigh your options and give you different viewpoints to consider while making the decision.

Treatment Using Donor Sperm

Once you've selected a sperm donor, treatment will proceed in the same manner as it would for a married couple, usually with intrauterine insemination (IUI) attempted first. The doctor will recommend either the use of medications, or what's known as a natural cycle in which no medication is used. Your own monthly cycle is monitored periodically through blood and ultrasound, or even the use of ovulation predictor kits at home. Once you are ready to ovulate, the sperm is introduced into the uterus with a special catheter.

In the event that unmedicated cycles are not successful after several tries, the doctor may recommend more aggressive therapies, like injectable medications or even in vitro fertilization (IVF).

Infertility Treatment for the Lesbian/ Gay Couple

It's not uncommon for lesbian/gay couples to want to start a family. This has traditionally been done through adoption, but thanks to the availability of third party reproduction, many gay and lesbian families are now electing to have their own, genetic children.

ALERT

It is highly recommended that you consult with an attorney who specializes in reproductive legal issues. He can help you make sense of the legal restrictions present in your state. Legal contracts need to be drafted in order to ensure that the ownership of the embryos remains with you and that there are no custody issues later on.

Lesbian Couples

A lesbian couple has several options when it comes to infertility treatment. One woman within the relationship must elect to carry the pregnancy. If there is a preference between partners, or a medical issue that prevents one of the partners from becoming pregnant, this should be factored into the decision-making process. If one of the partners is significantly older than the other, perhaps the younger partner should strongly consider carrying the pregnancy.

Treatment usually proceeds in the same manner as for a single woman: a sperm donor is selected, either known or anonymous, and a medical protocol is devised by the doctor.

Some couples elect to take a different approach: one partner acts as an egg donor, donating her eggs through IVF, which are then fertilized with the donated sperm. The resulting embryos are then transferred into the second partner. In essence, one partner contributes half of the genetics and the other partner carries the pregnancy.

Same-Sex Male Couples

Male couples have a trickier time when it comes to having their own child. One partner contributes the sperm, but an egg donor and gestational carrier are also needed. In most cases, IVF is the treatment of choice.

Some male couples elect to both contribute their sperm. The two samples are combined in the lab before fertilization, making it possible for either partner to be the genetic father of the child. If you choose, paternity testing can be done once the child is born.

Depending on the state where you live, there is most likely legislation dictating how surrogacy is regulated.

The couple can elect to use a known or unknown egg donor and carrier, or any combination in between. For example, they may want to use the sister of the partner who is not donating his sperm as the egg donor, but find a carrier through an agency. Or they may use an anonymous egg donor with a friend carrying the pregnancy. The decision is inherently personal and deserves a great deal of thought and consideration.

Where to Go from Here

After you've recognized that you may have a fertility problem, the next step is to go into a testing phase. Find a practitioner and program that you and your partner feel comfortable with. How many tests and what tests you and your partner need will be determined by your doctors who will base their diagnosis on medical records and how you respond to each individual test.

After the testing phase, you and your fertility team will sit down together with your partner and come up with a treatment plan. During the course of the treatment plan you will actively undergo therapies designed for you and your partner to increase your chances of conception. Pregnancy may be easily achieved once you and your partner have a diagnosis and are treated, or you may find that additional measures need to be taken as you progress through treatments. Both courses of action will be individually managed with your health care team.

Once you have made the decision to seek support, testing, and treatment of your fertility issues, you will likely have many questions. Finding answers to your questions may not be an easy road. However, it is not a road you will travel alone. Your partner and other family or friends you choose to confide in will help you along as you learn to take an active part in your medical care. You will learn how to be a good consumer of services and advocate for yourself.

Planning your family may have started when you were just a small child yourself. Perhaps you and your spouse have spent long nights picking out names for your future children, maybe even before you were married. Because of this, finding out that you or your partner suffers from infertility can be a devastating blow. Finding the right medical guide for you and your partner will be crucial to navigating the many options available. You will also need to build a support system to help hold you and be there to share your disappointments and ultimately your joys.

CHAPTER 2

Understanding Your Body

Remember high school biology? That week when you studied human reproduction and sat through the embarrassing lectures that you'd rather hear from anybody other than your high school science teacher? Well, that stuff is actually going to come in handy, and most likely, it's time for a review. Understanding how your body and reproduction works can make it easier to understand the infertility process.

Male Anatomy

The job of the male reproductive system is to produce sperm and deliver it into the female reproductive tract. Sperm cells hand down genes from generation to generation.

Every cell in the human body, except sperm and egg cells, contain forty-six chromosomes, the equivalent of two full copies of the human genetic code. It is the interaction of the two copies of the genome that produces the distinct characteristics people exhibit. Each sperm (and egg) cell carries only half of the forty-six chromosomes. When a sperm cell fertilizes an egg, the genetic material it contains combines with the egg's genetic material to create an embryo.

Sperm Production

In a normal healthy male, there is a complex process involved in making sperm. This process takes place in the testicles and is driven by the endocrine (hormonal) system. The hormones involved include some of the same hormones that play a role in your menstrual cycle, including luteinizing hormone (LH), follicle stimulating hormone (FSH), and gonadotropin releasing hormone (GnRH). The first two of those are produced in his pituitary gland, while GnRH is released by the male's hypothalamus, a tiny structure in the brain. Through a system of chemical messages from the GnRH, his body releases the FSH and LH, which in turn stimulates cells to begin producing testosterone. The testosterone and FSH facilitate the process of sperm production in the man's testes.

It takes about seventy-two days to create and mature a sperm cell (spermatozoa). Each sperm is made up of three essential parts: the head, the midpiece, and the tail. Sperm require a cooler environment than our body temperature to survive; therefore, they are housed in a man's scrotum, which hangs just outside of his body.

The Scrotum

The scrotum is an external sac located just behind the penis and contains the testicles, the two small organs that produce sperm. One of the scrotum's main functions is to regulate the temperature of the testicles. The sperm cells are very sensitive to changes in temperature, so it is important to keep the temperature as regular as possible. If the man's body becomes too warm, the scrotum will relax and lower the testicles away from the excess body heat. If the testicles are too cool, the scrotum will tense up and pull closer to the body.

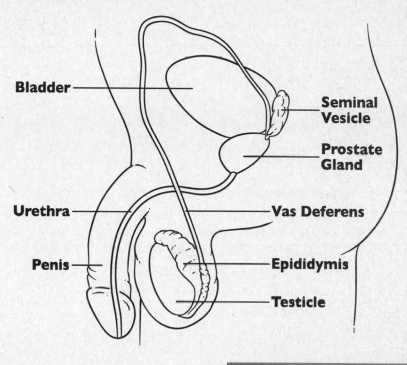

The male reproductive system

The Penis

Sperm cells pass from the testicles, where they're made, into the body where they pass through several small glands, including the prostate. These glands secrete fluids that are added to the sperm to create a mixture called semen. This fluid contains special proteins and chemicals that contribute to the survival of the sperm cells while they are in the female reproductive tract. The semen will eventually make its way out of the body as ejaculate. At each ejaculation, be it from sex or masturbation, between 20 and 200 million sperm are released.

Many people think of the penis as the main male organ of reproduction. Its job is to penetrate the female partner and deliver sperm from the scrotum to the inside of her body. The penis is rich in blood vessels and spongy tissue that, when sexually aroused, fill with blood and cause the penis to harden, making penetration possible.

FACT

Sperm will build up if a man doesn't ejaculate for a long period of time. Some of the built-up sperm will die away and be reabsorbed in the man's body, and some will be washed away as he urinates. This buildup of sperm isn't harmful to a man in any way, nor will it affect future fertility.

Another branch of the urethra carries urine from the bladder to the outside of the body, through the same opening, or meatus, as the sperm. There is a special valve that prevents urine from exiting the bladder when he is sexually aroused.

Female Anatomy

The job of the female reproductive system is to prepare for and carry a pregnancy to term. Each month, an egg is produced that will, if fertilized by a sperm cell, contribute half of the woman's genetic information to the resulting embryo. Her body will support, nourish, and protect the fetus for nine months, until the baby is able to survive on its own. Once ready, the body works to expel the baby from the woman's body.

External Anatomy

The vulva is the collective term for all of the external structures in the female reproductive system. There are two openings found within the vulva: the urethra and the vaginal opening. The urethra is the opening more toward the front of the body that is used to expel urine from the bladder. The vaginal opening is behind the urethra and leads into the reproductive system. It is the orifice that receives the penis during intercourse, and

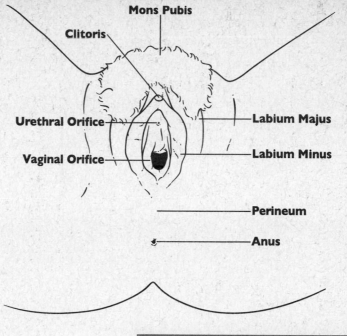

Mons Pubis

Clitoris

Urethral Orifice

Vaginal Orifice

Labium Majus

Labium Minus

Perineum

Anus

External female reproductive anatomy

through which a woman menstruates. During childbirth, the baby is delivered from the uterus through the vaginal canal.

Both openings are surrounded by protective tissue called the labia. There are two layers of labia: the thick outer labia majora whose outer side is covered with pubic hair, and the labia minora, which are inside of the labia majora. The labia minora are thinner, pink, and very sensitive. Within the two labia are small glands that secrete special lubricants to help facilitate intercourse.

The Vagina, Cervix, and Uterus

The cervix is the opening that connects the vagina to the uterus. It is a small tubular structure with two openings. Each opening is called an "os"—the external os is the one between the vagina and the cervix, and the internal os is between the cervix and the uterus. The cervix dilates during childbirth to allow passage of the baby into the birth canal. It is important for a woman to have routine pap smears, a test that checks the cervix for abnormal cells. These abnormal cells can be precursor to cervical cancer.

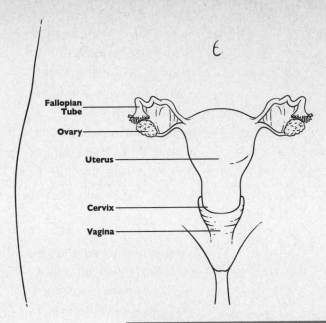

The internal female reproductive system

The uterus is a pear shaped, hollow, muscular organ in the lower abdomen. Every month, a relatively thick lining of blood and tissue develops on the inside surface of the uterine wall in order to support a pregnancy should one occur.

FACT

The lining of the uterus is called the endometrium. It is not just blood, as is commonly thought, but rather a collection of specialized, well-vascularized (rich in blood vessels) tissue that changes over the course of the month in response to hormones.

If pregnancy does not occur, the lining is shed during a woman's period, and a new lining is built up the following month.

The Ovaries and Fallopian Tubes

The ovaries are two small organs, each the size of a small grape, located in the lower pelvis on each side of the uterus. Each contains millions of immature eggs, which have been there since the woman was born;

no new eggs are ever made in the female body. This means that, if a woman is twenty-nine, her eggs are also twenty-nine years old. This is why older women are much more likely to have a child with Down's syndrome or other genetic issue; the older the eggs are, the more likely that some of the genetic material in the egg has degraded.

Once an egg, or oocyte, has been released at ovulation, it gets swept into the Fallopian tubes, two small tubes that connect to the uterus. The egg gets pushed down the length of the tube by little fingerlike projections called cilia that beat back and forth, moving the egg down the tube.

ALERT

If the Fallopian tubes become blocked, the egg can't travel down to the uterus, nor can the sperm travel into the tube, thus preventing fertilization and pregnancy. Blockages can occur in the tubes for a number of reasons, like infection, a previous ectopic pregnancy, or tubal damage from abdominal or pelvic surgery.

If fertilization were to occur, it would happen in the Fallopian tube. Once the egg reaches the uterus—about four to five days after ovulation—it is too late for fertilization to take place. If pregnancy does not occur, the egg is shed with the rest of the uterine lining as a period.

The Menstrual Cycle

Girls are born with about two million oocytes, or eggs. By the time a girl reaches puberty, she only has about 400,000 eggs left. A young girl's first period is called menarche and occurs on average around age twelve. Of course, there is great variation, as some girls start menstruating earlier while others won't begin until as late as age sixteen or seventeen.

The cessation of menses is a process called menopause, which typically happens around age fifty. As you reach menopause, the end of the fertile phase of your life, you will have very few eggs left. During the course of your fertile periods, you will have only produced about 400 mature eggs. The years leading up to menopause are called perimenopause and can start up to ten years before the last period.

The average length of a menstrual cycle—which is measured from the start of one period to the start of the next—is twenty-eight days, but it can be as short as twenty-one days and as long as thirty-five days. When you start to think about attempting to conceive a child, it can be helpful to track your cycles. Record the start date, how long the period is, and anything that you are concerned about. There are four stages of the menstrual cycle: the follicular, ovulatory, and luteal phases, and menstruation.

The Follicular Phase

The follicular phase is the beginning part of the cycle, when a follicle and the egg inside it begins to mature. The process begins when a special

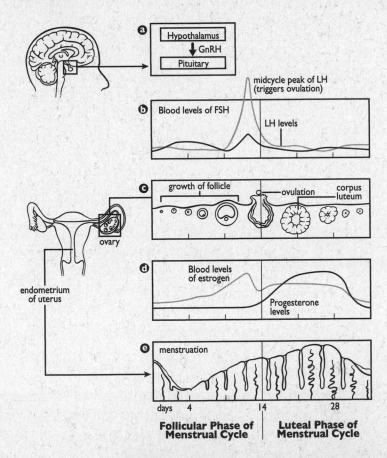

The hormone profile during the menstrual cycle

hormone, called gonadotropin-releasing hormone, is released from the hypothalamus. That hormone does exactly what its name implies—it causes gonadotropins to be released from the pituitary gland, another small gland in the brain. These gonadotropins, called follicle stimulating hormone (FSH) and lutenizing hormone (LH), stimulate follicular growth in the ovaries.

As the follicle develops, it secretes small amounts of a form of estrogen, called beta-estradiol, until the egg reaches maturity. At that point, the pituitary starts pumping out large amounts of LH, a surge that precedes ovulation by approximately thirty-six hours. Ovulation predictor kits work by detecting these elevated levels of LH.

Ovulation

Ovulation, or the release of a mature egg from the ovary, occurs approximately fourteen days into a cycle. Every cycle is different though, and you may ovulate on day sixteen one month and day thirteen the next. For that reason, it can be helpful to start testing for your LH surge a few days earlier then you expect ovulation to take place if you are using an ovulation predictor kit. You don't want to start too late and miss your surge.

The empty egg follicle is now known as the "corpus luteum" and it produces a hormone called progesterone.

ALERT

If you are consistently getting positive results on your ovulation predictor kit, even if it doesn't make sense that you'd be ovulating, it may be a sign of polycystic ovary syndrome (PCOS). Women with PCOS sometimes have persistently elevated levels of LH in their system. If this happens to you, make sure to speak with your doctor.

Contrary to popular belief, your ovaries do not necessarily take turns ovulating. In fact, some women will always ovulate from one ovary. Which ovary is chosen each month depends on where the dominant follicle resides. The ovary with the dominant follicle is the lucky one to release an egg that month.

You may be able to tell when you are ovulating without charting your menstrual cycle. Some women report feeling a small pain or cramp on one side or the other as the egg is released. This is called "mittelschmerz."

The Luteal Phase

The luteal phase is the second half of the cycle and is characterized by the presence of the corpus luteum (empty egg follicle) that produces large amounts of progesterone, the primary hormone of pregnancy in case of a possible pregnancy. If pregnancy does happen, eventually the placenta will take over as the progesterone producer and the corpus luteum will degenerate. The levels of progesterone in the body will wane if pregnancy does not occur, and it is this falling progesterone level that triggers the next menstrual period.

While all of these changes are occurring with the egg, the uterine lining is undergoing several changes as well. The lining is growing progressively thicker and becoming more developed in anticipation of the implantation of a fertilized egg.

Menstruation

If an embryo does not implant, the body sheds the uterine lining, expelling the blood, tissue, and egg as menses, or a woman's period. Hormone levels return to their baseline level and prepare for the start of the next cycle. Gonadotropin-releasing hormone is produced by the hypothalamus and the cycle starts again.

ESSENTIAL

Your clinic will ask you about the first day of your period. This typically means the first day that you have a full flow period, not counting any staining or spotting that happens before. If the full flow starts after 9:00 P.M., the next day is usually counted as day one. Clarify with your nurses if you have any questions.

▼ **TABLE 2-1: HORMONAL LEVELS DURING THE PHASES OF THE MENSTRUAL CYCLE**

Hormone	Follicular Phase	Ovulation	Luteal Phase	Menstrual Phase
Estradiol	Increases	Falls	Low	Low
FSH	Increases	Falls	Low	Low
LH	Increases	Peaks	Low	Low
Progesterone	Low	Starts to Rise	Peaks	Low

Summary of the hormonal changes during the menstrual cycle.

It's All about Timing

You probably knew that sex for procreation is about timing. When you're trying to conceive there are benefits to timing intercourse; the key is getting the timing right.

Now that you understand the mechanics of ovulation and your cycle, you will know what day you are mostly likely to ovulate. That is the day you are shooting for to fertilize that egg. However, this does not mean that you must have sex on that day.

Remember that the egg is viable for between twelve and twenty-four hours. Sperm can live, however, for much longer in your reproductive tract. You will want to ensure that you have live sperm attempting to reach your egg when you ovulate. You will want to have intercourse before, during, and after ovulation to accomplish this and ensure that all of your bases are covered.

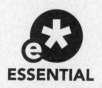

ESSENTIAL

Even in healthy men, sperm count can be lowered by excessive ejaculation. It does not matter how the ejaculation takes place. Masturbation or oral, vaginal, or anal sex can all lead to a decreased sperm count. During the time of month you are ovulating, it's best to wait twenty-four to thirty-six hours between ejaculations.

If you typically ovulate on day twelve of your cycle, you'll want to cover your bases by having intercourse on days eight, ten, twelve, fourteen, and sixteen. This ensures that the day of ovulation is covered, even if you've miscalculated the actual ovulation date.

Notice that you are not having sex every day in the previous example. Having intercourse every day can be detrimental to your goals of achieving a pregnancy. Your partner's sperm count will be lower the more often he ejaculates, so it is recommended that you have sex only every other day to give him a break.

Why do you need to have intercourse on so many days surrounding your ovulation date? You include the days before your cycle to ensure that sperm is present around the egg when it is released. You include the day of ovulation for perfect timing. Then you include the days after your intended day of ovulation to give the sperm another chance to get to the egg before it dies.

Sex Truths and Myths

There are an awful lot of old wives' tales out there regarding sex and conception, and not all of them are true. Knowing what's true and what's false can help you when trying to get pregnant.

Can You Influence the Gender According to When You Have Sex?

Each sperm carries one half of the genetic material of the man, and this is true of the sex chromosomes as well. Because males have both an X and a Y chromosome, one of the distinguishing characteristics of males, about half of the sperm carry the X chromosome while the other half carry the Y chromosome.

Females, on the other hand, have two X chromosomes. This means that every egg the woman produces should have an X chromosome as well. When one sperm cell fertilizes an egg, the egg contributes the X, and the sperm contributes either the X or the Y, depending on which chromosome it carries. If the sperm carries an X, the baby will be a girl because it now has two X chromosomes. If the sperm carries the Y, the baby will be a boy because the embryo will have an X and a Y chromosome.

It is thought that sperm carrying the Y swim faster but are less hearty then sperm carrying the X chromosome. Sperm carrying the X chromosome are thought to be stronger and slower. This is the basis for the belief that the Y carrying sperm will get to the egg quicker if you have sex right before or after ovulation. However, if you have sex a few days before ovulation, the Y carrying sperm should, in theory, die quicker, allowing the X carrying sperm to get to the egg once ovulation does occur.

Regardless of the gossip, studies have not proven this to be either true or false. There are some people who swear by the method and others who have disproven it within their own families. Whether or not it's true, it can't hurt to try!

Can You Get Pregnant If You Have Sex During Your Period?

Yes. The short answer is that it is always *possible*, though there are times, like when you have your period, when pregnancy is less likely to occur. You should always take precautions if you are not prepared for a pregnancy.

The shorter the time between your cycles is, the more likely it is that you will be ovulating shortly after your period finishes. Ovulation should occur fourteen days before your next period. This means that if you have twenty-three days between your cycles, ovulation is usually occurring around day nine. If your period is seven days long and you have sex on the last day, it is possible for sperm to be in your reproductive tract around the time the egg is released.

ALERT

If you notice that your cycles have consistently short luteal phases, that is if the time period from the day you detect your ovulation until you get your next period is frequently less than thirteen days, mention it to your doctor. This can indicate a luteal phase deficiency where the endometrium has not developed sufficiently.

Can You Get Pregnant If the Woman Is on Top?

Yes, you can get pregnant in any position. However, because you are upright, gravity may work against you by keeping some sperm from reaching the uterus. In most circumstances, this will not affect your chances of getting pregnant. If the male partner has an issue with his sperm count, you might want to consider a different position. The missionary position or even hands and knees can be the best positions for conception. Any position that allows for deeper penetration (it puts the sperm closer to the cervix) and keeps the woman lying down to prevent sperm from leaking out is optimal. Be creative!

Can You Get Pregnant If You Are a Virgin?

Again, yes. You can get pregnant even this is your first ovulation. As long as there is an egg cell that can be fertilized by a sperm cell, pregnancy can occur.

You Can't Get Pregnant If the Woman Has an Orgasm

Thankfully, this is just a myth! Studies have actually shown the opposite; that a woman's orgasm is quite important to the conception process. When a woman has an orgasm, a series of uterine and cervical contractions helps to pull sperm through the cervix and into the uterus. So go ahead and enjoy!

Basic Embryology

Embryology is the study of the beginning stages of human development during the early phases of pregnancy. It is a complex science that you don't need to know too much about, but there are a few concepts to understand that can help make going through treatment a little easier.

Fertilization

Fertilization usually takes place in the Fallopian tube and is the process where a single sperm cell penetrates the egg. Only one sperm cell can penetrate an egg.

As the sperm encounters the cells that surround the egg, special enzymes secreted by the sperm begin to break down those cells. The sperm will then encounter the zona pellucida, which you can compare to the shell of an egg. This is a very important step because a reaction occurs as the sperm penetrates the zona that makes the zona impenetrable to other sperm cells. The maternal chromosomes and paternal chromosomes begin to undergo

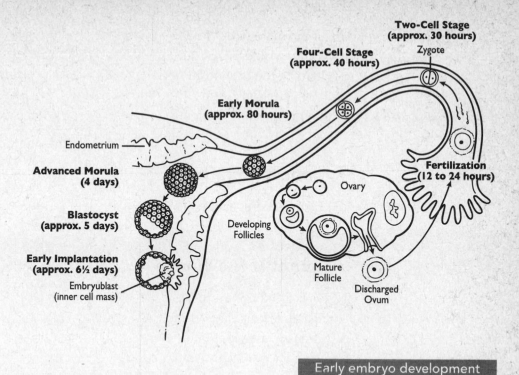

Early embryo development

a series of changes that eventually combines the genetics of the two cells (egg and sperm) into a single, unified genetic code. The two cells are now a single-celled zygote.

Over the next several days, the zygote begins a series of rapid divisions, into two cells, then four, then eight, etc. Around day three, it becomes a morula; a two-layered spherical structure with twelve to thirty-two cells. Until this point the zygote is still in the Fallopian tube.

FACT

Sometimes multiple sperm cells do fertilize an egg. This is usually a result of a defect in either the sperm or the egg. The pregnancy will not continue because of the severity of the impact on the fetus. If this is happening to you, it can't be diagnosed unless directly observed in the lab.

Around day four, the morula enters the uterus and starts to turn into a blastocyst. A small amount of fluid enters the morula from the uterus and begins separating the two layers of cells. The inner layer of cells, called the inner cell mass, will eventually become the fetus. The thin, outer layer of cells, called the outer cell mass, will become the placenta.

Implantation

The blastocyst will float around in the uterus for approximately two days while it forms. The zona pellucida begins to disintegrate and disappear, allowing the blastocyst to rapidly grow in size. This is called hatching of the blastocyst.

FACT

In some women, usually older women, the zona pellucida is thickened, making it difficult for the blastocyst to hatch. If the blastocyst hasn't hatched, it cannot implant in the uterine wall. A thickened zona can only be diagnosed when the embryologist notices it in the lab during IVF.

Six days after fertilization the blastocyst will burrow into the uterine lining, a process known as implantation. The implanted blastocyst will undergo a number of changes as the cells begin to differentiate into not only the developing embryo, but the extra embryonic structures including the placenta, yolk sac, and amniotic cavity. At the end of this week, the pregnancy will start to produce a hormone called human chorionic gonadotropin, or hCG, that will continue to support the pregnancy and the corpus luteum. This will keep the corpus luteum producing abundant amounts of progesterone, which will in turn also support the pregnancy.

Early Pregnancy Testing

Up until this point, the woman will not know that she is pregnant. At the end of the second week of development, around four weeks past her last menstrual period, the levels of hCG will be detectable in her blood and urine. This is right around the time she may miss a menstrual period, prompting her to take a pregnancy test.

Home pregnancy tests work by checking for the presence of hCG in your urine. You place a few drops of urine onto the test strip, and the drops are filtered through special paper that has been treated with chemicals that can detect any hCG present. If the hormone is present, the pregnancy test is positive. Exactly how this will be indicated on your testing kit will be explained in the instructions. Some tests will show two lines, whereas others have a dark circle or a plus sign.

ALERT

If you do not think you can actually urinate on the test stick for the given amount of time, try catching the urine in a clean paper cup. Then dip the test stick in the urine for the specified amount of time and follow the instructions from there.

Consumers beware! Not all urine pregnancy tests are created equally. The hormone is measured in mIU/mL (milli-international units per milliliter), and different tests will measure different amounts of hCG. There are tests that measure very small amounts of hCG—some as low as 20–25 mIU/mL—and other tests won't detect hCG until it reaches quantities that measure at least 250 mIU/mL. Remember that the lower the number, the sooner you'll know.

While these tests can accurately indicate a pregnancy based on the presence of hCG, there are often false negatives because not everyone will have the same amounts of hCG in their urine that early. If you've taken a home pregnancy test and it was negative, do not assume you are not pregnant. Wait a few days and try again; it's quite likely that you simply tested too early.

Understanding how you and your partner's bodies work, including when you ovulate, the length of your cycle, and other pieces of important information, is first step in your journey toward pregnancy. This knowledge can help aid in conception and also help you understand what is happening during your fertility treatment.

CHAPTER 3

Causes of Infertility

Experts estimate that 40 percent of couples with infertility have female factor infertility, 40 percent have male factor infertility, and 20 percent of couples suffer from unexplained infertility. Many couples have a combination of factors that may be keeping them from getting pregnant. A thorough evaluation will help your reproductive endocrinologist (RE) determine the cause(s) of your infertility.

Male Factor

Having male factor infertility can mean a variety of things, from a mild reduction in sperm count to a complete absence of sperm to the inability to ejaculate. If a man has anything that inhibits the production, movement, or ejaculation of sperm, that issue will prevent conception from occurring.

Abnormal Sperm

Oligospermia is the production of too little sperm. Clinically, oligospermia is defined as less than 20 million sperm per milliliter of semen. Only a test of the semen can determine this diagnosis. Azoospermia, a condition in which the man produces no sperm, is fairly uncommon, but it's a serious condition because men with no sperm are completely sterile without medical intervention. There are two categories of azoospermia: obstructive and nonobstructive. Nonobstructive azospermia is diagnosed when no sperm are produced by the testes at all, usually a result of genetic, hormonal, or congenital conditions. When sperm cells are produced, but are unable to be ejaculated because of blockages within the reproductive tract, this is known as obstructive azospermia. A vasectomy is one type of obstructive azospermia.

A normal sperm is shaped like a snake, with a long tail and an oval-shaped head. The sperm's shape actually helps it reach and eventually penetrate the egg. A deformity of any kind in the shape of the sperm can affect the quality of movement and the ability of the sperm to penetrate the egg.

Sperm is said to be low quality if there are problems with its shape. This can be a greater problem than having a low sperm count because it can prevent other treatments from being used. However, advances in the treatment of male factor infertility are growing and becoming more widely available.

Sperm that has difficulty is getting to the egg can also present problems to the couple trying to conceive. The movement of the sperm is called its "motility." The tail of the sperm moves and thrashes in a spiral-like motion to propel the sperm forward and toward the egg. Motility is said to be impaired if the sperm is unable to move through the cervical fluid, or if the sperm has problems with its ability to swim. This can be the result of a defective sperm or the result of a shape that is abnormal.

To fix a low sperm count, doctors can sometimes prescribe medications or even perform a procedure to directly retrieve sperm from the testicles. This sperm can then be used for other procedures, such as intracytoplasmic sperm injection (ICSI), in which the sperm is injected directly into the egg just before an in vitro procedure.

Varicocele

Some men suffer from a problem known as a varicocele, which is a collection of varicose veins located behind and above the testes. When a varicocele is present it restricts blood flow to and from the testes, causing a problem with swelling and with the temperature in the testicles. This heat can damage or kill the sperm and also damage the valves that regulate blood flow around the testes.

You may find a varicocele is in one or both testicles, though it is much more common to find the varicocele in the left testicle. A varicocele is not always an indication that the man is infertile; about 15 percent of men will have a varicocele, and it is the cause of male infertility in about 40 percent of the cases of male factor infertility. Varicoceles may form after injury to the scrotum or testicle, or they can be just a random occurrence.

FACT

Varicoceles are more common on the left testicle than the right, occurring in the left in about 85 percent of men who have varicoceles. It is hypothesized that this is because the left spermatic vein is longer. However, it is possible to have varicoceles on both sides. This occurs in about 20 percent of men with this problem.

Surgery may be one option if your partner suffers from varicoceles. This is usually done on an outpatient basis and offers one of the best chances to aid in conception. About 60 percent of men will be able to conceive with no additional treatment beyond surgery. Your partner should have a semen analysis repeated a few months after his surgery to recheck the quality and count of his sperm.

An important factor in the decision on whether to operate is the age of the female partner. Because it can take six months or longer for the full effect to be seen, delaying pregnancy may not be the best course of action when his partner is older or has issues with ovarian reserve.

Retrograde Ejaculation

Retrograde ejaculation can be a problem for men as well. In this situation, the neck of the bladder does not close properly and some or all of his semen is washed back into the bladder during ejaculation. In other words, the semen does not leave the penis through the urethra.

Cloudy urine after ejaculation can be one of the signs that your man suffers from retrograde ejaculation. You may also notice this if the quantity of semen has drastically changed over the years or after surgery to the bladder. It may also be caused by a structural defect the man has had since birth. Sometimes problems like diabetes can also be to blame for retrograde ejaculation.

Hormonal Problems

Hormonal checks and balances are a big part of male factor infertility. Just as the hormonal system for you must be perfectly in balance for everything to run smoothly, your partner's hormones are also very important. Small problems with hormone levels can create big problems with fertility. These are often tested for very early on in the process.

Genetic Conditions

The most common cause of lowered sperm counts is Klinefelter's syndrome, a genetic problem in which the man has an additional X chromosome (XXY instead of XY). This results in little or no sperm production because of the abnormal development of his testicles. He may also suffer from a decreased level of testosterone.

Another potential source of problems with male fertility is a situation in which the man's Y chromosome is missing some genetic material, called Y microdeletions, affecting his ability to produce sperm.

ESSENTIAL

Ask your physician if it is beneficial to have a genetic screening. This is a simple blood test to analyze the sex chromosomes to make sure that there is only one X and one Y. The lab can also check for Y microdeletions to make sure that a genetic issue is not the cause for your partner's low sperm count.

Other Factors Affecting the Sperm

There are a multitude of things that can affect your sperm, from infections to medications to certain chemicals you are exposed to in your daily life. Sometimes this effect is temporary, other times it could be long lasting. For example, having mumps as a child could damage the testicles, permanently destroying the ability of a man to produce sperm. But having the flu a few months back could also temporarily reduce the sperm that the man was making at that time.

Certain drugs, like marijuana and steroids, could also temporarily affect sperm count. Make sure to be honest with your doctor. The physician will not judge you, and having all of the information is an absolute necessity so the doctor can plan the appropriate care for you. Without it, unnecessary surgery or medication might be prescribed when all that is needed is to stop taking the offending drugs.

Ovulatory Disorders

Ovulation is a key step in getting pregnant, so anything that interferes with this process will make pregnancy difficult, or even impossible if ovulation does not occur all together. Anovulation means the complete absence of ovulation, while oligoovulation means irregular ovulation.

PCOS

In addition to estrogen and progesterone, women also produce hormones called androgens. Testosterone, the primary male hormone, is one type of androgen. Androgens are elevated in women with polycystic ovary syndrome, or PCOS, leading to irregular ovulation and symptoms like acne, obesity, abnormal hair growth on your face or chest (hirsutism), or even male pattern baldness.

ESSENTIAL

A medication called Metformin is often used to treat PCOS. While Metformin is not approved for use by the U.S. Food and Drug Administration (FDA) as a treatment for PCOS, it is thought to help correct the insulin resistance that many women with PCOS have. Many patients taking Metformin have reported that their menstrual cycles resume and they find a reduction in the severity of their symptoms.

While PCOS certainly affects your fertility and appearance, it also affects your body in a number of other ways. It is thought to decrease your body's response to insulin, which eventually leads to insulin resistance and diabetes. Additionally, women with PCOS are at greater risk for health problems like heart disease, high cholesterol, and high blood pressure.

Luckily, PCOS-related infertility is usually quite easy to treat. Medications like Clomid and forms of follicle stimulating hormone (FSH) are given to induce ovulation.

Premature Ovarian Failure

Another name for menopause is ovarian failure. Most women go through menopause in their forties or fifties, but sometimes women will start experiencing ovarian failure when they are significantly younger, even in their twenties or thirties. Symptoms include irregular menstrual cycles, changes in libido, vaginal dryness, and hot flashes.

Ovarian failure means that the number and quality of your eggs has decreased. This often comes as a surprise to young women who may not realize that they could be going through menopause at such a young age, especially since the cause of premature menopause is unknown. If you are diagnosed early enough, there may be enough time to try aggressive ovulation induction to help you achieve pregnancy with as little intervention as possible.

Women with premature ovarian failure typically do not respond well to the medication, including the high doses required during IVF treatment. If the ovarian failure has progressed to this point, your doctor may recommend that you use donated eggs.

FACT

Cancer treatments, like chemotherapy and radiation therapy, can also cause premature ovarian failure. If you have been diagnosed with cancer, it is important to discuss fertility preservation with your oncologist as soon as possible. There may be ways to preserve some level of fertility, or you may be able to freeze some eggs for use after treatment.

Uterine/Menstrual Conditions

A properly developed uterine lining is just as important to conceiving a child as is regular ovulation. The shape of your uterus is also important to achieving pregnancy; it can help direct the sperm to the Fallopian tubes. The fragile lining helps the fertilized egg find a new home and embed itself in the uterine lining. Any problems with this delicate balance and the fertility level falls.

Scarring of the Uterus

If you have experienced previous uterine surgeries for miscarriages, abortions, or a procedure known as dilatation and curettage (D&C), you may have potential scarring of the lining of the uterus. These scars, which may not be noticeable until you attempt to conceive, can cause you to have interruptions in your menstrual cycles. Though this is not a very common occurrence, it is possible so you'll need to report all surgeries to your physician so he has all the information necessary to make the correct diagnosis. Scar tissue within the uterine cavity is called Asherman's Syndrome. Asherman's Syndrome may cause amenorrhea and infertility.

Endometriosis

Endometriosis is tissue that looks and acts like the lining of the uterus but that grows elsewhere, usually in the abdomen. If you suffer from endometriosis, these tissues will grow and then bleed at the end of every normal menstrual cycle. Because the blood has no place to go, this can cause pain and swelling inside the abdomen or wherever the tissues are located.

QUESTION

I had an abortion in the past, and I really don't want to tell my doctor, should I?
Absolutely! It is very important to tell your physician about every surgery you have had, particularly as it relates to your reproductive tract. You may tell your physician without the presence of your partner if it makes you more comfortable. Your doctor will not be judgmental, but needs to know the medical facts to make the most correct diagnosis.

The most common symptom of endometriosis is painful menstrual cramps, though there may be other symptoms. The good news is that the amount of pain you feel is not necessarily relative to the amount of endometriosis you actually have. You may also experience pain in places like your intestines, if that's where the tissues are growing. Ironically, some women with endometriosis have no symptoms at all.

The only real way to diagnose endometriosis is to do exploratory surgery to see if tissues are growing. This is usually done with a minor surgical procedure, called laparoscopic surgery, which minimizes invasion into your body.

Endometriosis can cause scarring where the tissue grows, and it is most common to find endometriosis growing in or around the Fallopian tubes and ovaries. Scar tissues in these areas can create blockages of the Fallopian tubes or cause you to have difficulties with ovulation.

While endometriosis cannot be always identified as the cause of infertility, it can make your diagnosis more complicated. Endometriosis occurs more in women with fertility issues, and it gets worse with age. This condition is the suspected cause of about 15 percent of all cases of female infertility.

Fibroids

Fibroids are benign, i.e., noncancerous, growths in the smooth muscles of the uterus. The cause of fibroids is unknown; they can vary in number and size and may or may not cause symptoms, including abdominal/pelvic pain, difficult and painful periods, pelvic pressure, and infertility. They've also been implicated in recurrent pregnancy loss. If you are trying to get pregnant and a fibroid is discovered, the treatment of choice is usually surgical removal of the fibroid.

Amenorrhea

Amenorrhea is the lack of a menstrual cycle. You have primary amenorrhea if you have never had a menstrual cycle. If you have previously had regular menstrual cycles but have not had one for more than six months, you are said to be experiencing secondary amenorrhea. You may have had previously irregular cycles but have not had a menstrual cycle for twelve months—that is also known as secondary amenorrhea.

It's important to distinguish between the types of amenorrhea as the causes of the two are very different. Likewise, the testing and treatments for amenorrhea are different depending on whether you are suffering from the primary or secondary loss of your menstrual cycles.

Secondary amenorrhea is the more likely suspect of your fertility problem. Your amenorrhea can be caused by something as simple as the medication you are on. A complex issue related to your hormone production can also produce secondary amenorrhea. Testing by your healthcare practitioner will help determine the cause of your lack of menstrual cycle in about 85 percent of the cases.

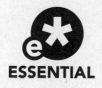

ESSENTIAL

Many women complain about lack of periods in the time immediately after they stop taking the pill, but this is usually something that will correct itself in time. Generally within the first six months of discontinuation, more than 99 percent of women will find that their periods return.

Hormonal imbalances are the most common cause of secondary amenorrhea. When prolactin levels are elevated, for example, then the other hormones necessary for keeping your cycle regular are thrown off kilter and your periods may stop.

There are other hormonal causes of secondary amenorrhea, including hypothyroidism and Cushing's syndrome. In hypothyroidism, your body doesn't produce enough of the thyroid hormones that can alter your periods. With Cushing's syndrome, your adrenal glands are overactive, and this causes hormonal fluctuations that prevent your menstrual cycles. Rapid weight loss can also be associated with the loss of your menstrual cycle, as losing a significant amount of weight or body fat in a short time can cause your body to stop ovulating. This is particularly a danger if you suffer from anorexia nervosa. Excessive amounts of exercise—marathon running, for example—can also alter your hormones enough to affect your fertility.

Hormonal Problems

Your hormones play an important role in the regulation of your menstrual cycle and fertility. But it's not just the reproductive hormones that are important. Abnormal levels of other hormones can have a dramatic effect on your fertility as well.

Hyperprolactinemia

Prolactin is a hormone secreted by the brain that promotes lactation. Hyperprolactinemia is an elevated amount of prolactin, a condition that can affect your ability to ovulate and menstruate normally. As with all other ovulatory disorders, this can make it difficult to get pregnant. The most common symptom of hyperprolactinemia is milk leaking from your breasts. Not everyone with hyperprolactinemia experiences this though.

Thyroid Disorders

Your thyroid gland produces hormones that are essential to the functioning of your entire body and general well-being. You can have problems with anovulation if certain thyroid hormones are elevated. This should be one of the primary hormones tested at your initial fertility evaluation.

Recurrent Pregnancy Loss

Having a miscarriage can be very difficult. Some couples have endured multiple miscarriages, and yet don't really have an explanation for why it keeps happening. Testing will sometimes reveal a reason for the losses, and other times it won't. The good news is that in most situations, there is still an excellent chance that you can have a healthy pregnancy.

Thrombophilias

A thrombophilia is an abnormality in the way that your blood clots. Normally this is not an issue, but it can play a role in your ability to maintain a pregnancy.

Thrombophilias are easily diagnosed through a simple blood test, called a thrombophilia panel. This panel is actually composed of a number of tests that look at the various components that make up the normal clotting cascade. And there are a lot of them!

If the test shows an abnormality, you may need to take a medication such as Metanx (which is a combination of B vitamins and folate) or Lovenox (a blood thinner) to help your body correct any clotting issues. Your doctor will advise you when and how long to take the medication. Often, correcting this underlying issue can give you a better prognosis for future pregnancies.

ALERT

If you experience a loss and require or are given the choice of a D&C, a surgical procedure to remove the pregnancy, make sure to request that the genetics of the specimen are analyzed. This can help give your physician insight into why the loss happened.

Genetics

Having a miscarriage is nature's way of preventing dangerous genetic mutations from entering the human genome. In fact, chromosomal abnormalities are the most common cause for miscarriage. In most cases the abnormality is just a fluke and not evidence of a deeper genetic issue, but it is important to rule that out as a cause. Your doctor will probably check you and your partner's karyotype to make sure that you have the correct number and type of sex chromosomes (i.e., Xs and Ys).

Your physician may also check one or both of you to determine if either of you carry the gene for certain genetic diseases. This is to ensure that you don't inadvertently pass on a severe illness to your child that might have otherwise been prevented.

Uterine Abnormalities

Abnormalities of the uterus can be something that you're born with, like a double uterus or a uterus that is divided by a wall (septate). Some women also have problems with fibroids, growths that can occur any place in the uterus. The good news is that the majority of these problems can be dealt with prior to conception through surgery, thus increasing your chances of a healthy pregnancy.

Tubal Factor

Your Fallopian tubes play a vital role in your fertility. Without them, or if they are blocked, the egg is not able to meet up with the sperm. The most common cause of tubal blockages is infections and trauma. Sexually transmitted infections, like chlamydia and gonorrhea, are frequent culprits because they can cause scarring within the tube itself.

Trauma is the other major cause of tubal scarring. Ectopic pregnancies (pregnancies that implant in the Fallopian tube), endometriosis, and even surgery can all cause damage to tissues in the Fallopian tubes. A ruptured appendix, bowel obstructions, or other type of pelvic surgery can also lead to blockages in the tubes or inflammation that creates a thickened lining. Remember, any thickening of the tubes' lining can create a potential problem for the egg or sperm.

It is also possible to be born with congenital problems of the Fallopian tubes. This can mean that your tubes are blocked, incomplete, or missing due to some genetic fluke prior to your birth. Treatment options for all tubal issues include surgery and/or IVF.

Unexplained Infertility

Perhaps one of the most frustrating diagnoses is unexplained infertility. Even with all the testing that is available to couples today, there will be cases where doctors cannot determine the source of the infertility. The reasons for unexplained infertility vary widely, but many couples will suffer from a source that no one can explain. If you have been given a diagnosis of unexplained infertility, you may feel like nothing can be done to help you. This is not true.

While the cause of your infertility is not known, many practitioners will begin treatments starting with the basics. By attempting the less complicated fertility treatments and advancing toward the higher end of that scale, you will certainly be given every chance of conceiving. Sometimes in the course of treatment, usually IVF, the embryologist will notice something that may give some sort of an explanation. Some examples include a thickened zona, which prevents hatching of the blastocyst, or the failure of any of the eggs to fertilize. For this reason, some infertility doctors will recommend IVF as a diagnostic tool. You may or may not agree with this approach; in fact, some couples opt to continue trying to conceive naturally or opt for other methods of creating a family.

Whatever the cause of your infertility, having a clear picture of what is going on will help your RE treat you more effectively. It's not uncommon for the testing phase to last several weeks, or even a few months, as the specialist narrows down what the problem may be.

CHAPTER 4

Preparing for Infertility Treatment

Once you've made the decision to seek out the advice of an infertility specialist, a multitude of questions often come up. What should we do to prepare? Should my partner avoid alcohol? Can we have sex? Can I continue to exercise? Can I take over-the-counter medications? These questions are very common and knowing the answers can help make a frightening process less so.

Maintaining a Healthy Weight

It's no secret that the United States is facing an obesity crisis. There are many physicians that refuse to discuss a patient's weight with her, but this is a great disservice to the patient. If your physician mentions that weight loss should be a priority for you, she is not being mean. Being overweight makes pregnancy, labor, and delivery significantly more difficult. Additionally, carrying extra weight increases you and your baby's risk for complications like gestational diabetes and preeclampsia.

Determining Your Healthy Weight

Essentially, you want your weight to be within the normal body mass index (BMI) range. BMI compares your height and weight to analyze the amount of body fat you have. It's easy to calculate using tools that you can find online. Check out *www.nhlbisupport.com/bmi*, a calculator designed by the U.S. Department of Health and Human Services. Simply enter your height and weight and click on "compute BMI" to see your results.

A healthy BMI is between 18.5 and 24.9. A BMI below 18.4 is considered underweight, a BMI between 25.0 and 29.9 is considered overweight, and someone with one above 30 is considered to be obese. Try to not get caught up in the numbers though. If your BMI is 25.1 and you exercise regularly and eat a fairly healthy diet, perhaps try to eliminate some of the extra sugar and fat in your diet and incorporate a little extra exercise. This slightly higher number does not mean that you should not try to get pregnant until your BMI is below 24.9.

However, if you find that your BMI is in the high overweight to obese range, you might want to consider holding off on pregnancy until you can get your weight down into a healthier range.

Weight Loss During or Before Infertility Treatment

Let's face it. There are an abundance of weight loss plans and strategies out there. Look around on the Internet or even on the shelves at your local book store, and chances are you'll find at least a dozen books and plans promising to deliver easy weight loss. Do yourself a favor and ignore them all. Weight loss is hard work and takes effort, and it is best achieved through lasting lifestyle changes. Most of the diets promising "quick results" will deliver just that, but then you'll likely regain the weight once you stop following the plan.

The basic principle of weight loss is that you need to burn more calories through cardiovascular exercise and weight training than you are eating. The first step is to honestly evaluate your lifestyle. Are you active or do you lead a sedentary lifestyle? Keep a food journal in which you track the amount of calories, fat, protein, and carbohydrates you eat over a week or two. Record everything you put in your mouth, including every "bite," "taste," and "piece." Chances are you'll be surprised by what you are actually eating over the course of the week. Use the results to guide your future decisions.

QUESTION

Are there places online where I can track my calories and exercise? Yes. Check out *www.sparkpeople.com* and *www.caloriecount.about.com* for free diet and exercise trackers. They can be useful for both short-term food journaling, or for losing weight in the long term as well.

If you choose to go the route of an organized diet plan, Weight Watchers is your best option. They stress portion control and healthy lifestyle changes, which are essential skills for long-term success.

Getting Control over Your Diet

Remember the food pyramid? It's a great place to start! By eating more whole grains, fruits, vegetables, dairy, and lean protein, and sparingly consuming fatty and sugary foods, you'll take the first steps on your way to good health. Ideally, you'll have four servings of vegetables per day and three servings of fruits.

Remember that variety is important when eating healthy as it ensures that you get many different vitamins and minerals every day. It also helps prevent you from becoming bored with your new eating habits. You should eat fresh fruits and vegetables whenever possible. The closer they are from where they came (be the vine or the ground), the better they are for you. Grazing, or eating smaller, more frequent meals, can help you achieve the variety you need in healthy amounts. This can also help balance out blood sugar problems.

Protein is the building block of every cell in your body and the body of your baby-to-be. Remember that the prenatal period up through your baby's first birthday is the period of most rapid growth for babies' brains. It's important to get plenty of protein to aid in this development.

Pregnant women should get at least 75 grams of protein a day. It can help prevent illness during pregnancy like eclampsia or toxemia. You will require more protein if you are expecting twins, if you are younger, and in some other specific situations, all of which your doctor will advise you.

Don't worry if you follow a vegan or vegetarian diet; there are many plant-based protein sources that you can choose from. Eggs, egg whites, and reduced fat dairy products are great options for the vegetarian, while soy products, beans, and nuts/nut butters are appropriate for everyone. Don't forget whole grains, either: Quinoa and Israeli couscous have five or six grams of protein per serving.

FACT

A printout of the food pyramid is a great tool to keep on your refrigerator for reference. Keeping a copy handy and even using it as a checklist can help keep you on track as you master this new style of healthy eating. You can find it online at *www.mypyramid.gov/mypyramid/index.aspx.*

Eating a healthy diet doesn't mean you have to completely give up fast food or chocolate cake. It simply means that you base your nutritional standards on foods that help grow a healthy baby. Anything that falls outside of this standard should be consumed only occasionally in addition to your regular foods. Having dessert or splurging on a greasy pizza once in a while isn't going to hurt your chances of having a healthy baby.

If you have special dietary needs, consider seeing a dietician. This is particularly great for you if you suffer from an eating disorder, diabetes, anemia (low iron), or other nutritional problems. Your doctor or midwife should be able to make a referral.

Plenty of Water

Water, water, everywhere! Now is the ideal time to get into the water habit. You need to consume at least six to eight 8-ounce glasses of water per day. Not only will this help rid your body of toxins, but it will also help keep you well hydrated. During pregnancy, staying well hydrated can make your skin more elastic and healthy, help with the prevention of stretch marks, and help decrease your risk of preterm labor.

Try drinking water throughout the day. Keep in mind that if you're thirsty, you've waited too long to drink! Your cells and tissues are already depleted of water before your body registers thirst. Drinking water regularly will help keep your body balanced.

Vitamins

Prenatal vitamins can be very important to ensuring you get the vitamins and minerals you need. Vitamins are not meant to replace the foods you eat. Rather, they should complement the food you eat. Your prenatal vitamins should be taken as directed by your practitioner.

Folate, or folic acid, is an absolute necessity for women who are trying to conceive. Taking folic acid prior to pregnancy has recently been shown to be much more beneficial than starting once a pregnancy has occurred. You need 400 micrograms of folic acid every day when trying to conceive, and 600 micrograms each day once you are pregnant; this will help prevent neural tube defects, like spina bifida and anencephaly. It is readily found in vitamins sold over-the-counter or by prescription. It is also found in some fortified foods like cereals and grains.

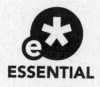

ESSENTIAL

Not all vitamins are created equally. It is possible for you to get too much of certain vitamins, such as vitamin A, which can cause birth defects if taken in large quantities. Be sure to show any vitamin supplement to your practitioner prior to taking it during pregnancy.

Guidelines for Exercise

Exercise is a healthy addition for almost everyone. It is important to discuss with your doctor whether it is healthy for you to continue exercising throughout fertility treatment and pregnancy. Make sure to clarify if there are any particular forms or types of exercise that you should refrain from. For example, your physician may say that all forms of cardio are fine, but to avoid any kind of weight training that puts pressure on your lower abdomen.

If you exercise regularly and get the go ahead from your doctor, feel free to continue. If you do not currently exercise, now is a great time to get started. Take it slowly by just adding in extra activity throughout your day. For example, try walking instead of taking the car when you go shopping. If you must drive, park in the farthest parking spot from the store you are going to.

FACT

When first starting out, try wearing a pedometer, a small tool that you wear on your clothes that counts the number of steps you take. You can purchase one at any major sports store for under $30. Aim for a minimum of 10,000 steps per day.

Any type of exercise will do. You should aim to do your exercising for about thirty minutes nearly every day of the week and, these don't have to be the same exercises all the time. Learn to incorporate exercise into your healthy lifestyle. For example, can you walk to the library? Perhaps you could ride your bike to work. Look for ways to make exercise fit in to your daily routine.

Behavioral Changes

Perhaps the most common questions asked by new moms-to-be is "is this safe?" Most women entering this time in their lives are more aware then anyone of how the things they put into their body will affect their baby and fertility. In general, the same rules apply when first trying to conceive and going through infertility treatment as in pregnancy.

Alcohol

You probably know that pregnant women should avoid alcohol. By learning to decline a glass of wine with your dinner during the preconception phase, you will be mentally preparing yourself for this lifestyle change when you are actually pregnant. Add an extra glass of water to your diet in place of alcohol, and try sparkling waters or juices to add some variety.

What this means is that you need to think long and hard about each glass of alcohol you drink. Where are you in your cycle? Could you already be pregnant and not know it yet? How would you feel about this glass of alcohol if the pregnancy test turned positive in a week? Would it worry you? If the answer is yes, don't drink it.

Alcohol is dangerous to your growing baby in many ways. It can cause brain damage, mental retardation, growth deformities, and other problems depending on how much you drank and the point you were in your cycle when you drank it. The first three to eight weeks of pregnancy, before you usually know you're pregnant, are the most critical in terms of not drinking.

ALERT

Don't think that because you aren't pregnant yet that you are off the hook. It's not unheard of for a woman to become pregnant at certain points throughout your infertility cycle (i.e., before your pregnancy test) or even naturally in between cycles. Besides, you'll want your health and fertility to be optimal before cycling.

Fetal alcohol syndrome (FAS) is a serious disorder caused by drinking during pregnancy, and it is unknown how much it takes to cause a child to suffer from this serious disease. Research shows that having seven or more drinks a week, or even a single occasion of binge drinking (five or more drinks at once), during your pregnancy puts your baby at risk. Another related problem that has shown up recently is called fetal alcohol effects (FAE), and it is believed that this is caused by lesser amounts of alcohol. It is best not to drink at all, since researchers and doctors don't know conclusively how much is too much.

If you have a serious problem with alcohol, there are many places you can get help. Some programs are designed specifically to help women who are pregnant or planning to become pregnant quit drinking. It's never too early to start.

Nicotine and Smoking

Smoking and other forms of tobacco are harmful to your baby-to-be as well. The sooner you stop smoking, the greater your chances are for a healthy pregnancy. Smoking during pregnancy can increase the risks of:

- **Premature birth:** Being born premature is the leading cause of neonatal death. It also increases the potential for problems with learning disabilities, mental retardation, and other problems.
- **Placenta previa:** When the placenta covers parts or your entire cervix, you and your baby are at a greater risk of death from hemorrhage. This condition also necessitates a Cesarean delivery for the birth.
- **Placental abruption:** An abruption of the placenta occurs when the placenta tears off the wall of the uterus. If not delivered immediately, the baby will die and you may hemorrhage as well.
- **Breathing problems:** Both immediately after birth and throughout life, breathing problems like asthma are greater in children whose parents smoked during pregnancy or in children who are exposed to secondhand smoke soon after they are born.
- **General illness:** Babies of smokers are more likely to have ear infections and upper respiratory infections, and are at a greater risk of dying from sudden infant death syndrome (SIDS).

It's estimated that about 426,000 women smoke during pregnancy every year—that's about 13 percent of all pregnant women, according to the American Legacy Foundation. This organization has created a program to help pregnant women and women planning to become pregnant to stop smoking. You can call them at 1-866-66START or visit *www.americanlegacy.org/greatstart*.

Smoking during pregnancy and exposing your child to secondhand smoke are very serious matters. It is in your best interest, and that of your baby-to-be, that you quit smoking in the planning phases. It's also helpful if your partner quits with you. Soon, you'll find even your health is better!

Caffeine's Common Effects

Caffeine is one of those chemicals that most people do not consider to be a drug even though it is a powerful stimulant. It can be found in many drinks like coffee and soft drinks, and now you can even buy bottled water laced with caffeine. Caffeine increases your blood flow and can make you feel wide-awake and alert.

Since there is no recommended daily allowance (RDA) of caffeine, it's hard to set a limit. Most practitioners will tell you that it's okay to have 100mg of caffeine each day, which is roughly equivalent to one 8-ounce cup a day of your favorite caffeinated product. Decaffeinated coffees or teas are a great alternative as well.

Over-the-Counter Medications and Supplements

You should never assume that just because something is available over-the-counter that it is safe for you to take. This rule holds especially true when you're pregnant and when you're going through infertility treatment. Even something as seemingly benign as ibuprofen can affect your uterine lining and may be unsafe in early pregnancy.

ESSENTIAL

Although you should definitely speak with your doctor, acetaminophen is generally accepted to be safe during both infertility treatment and early pregnancy, and is helpful for most aches and pains. Acetaminophen is also usually preferable to other drugs like ibuprofen and naproxen.

Medications are rated in pregnancy categories on a scale from A to X. Drugs that are labeled as A or B are safe to take when pregnant. Drugs labeled with a C are acceptable based on whether the benefits of taking the drug outweigh the risk of not taking it. According to the FDA, class C drugs indicate that "adequate, well-controlled human studies are lacking, and animal studies have shown a risk to the fetus or are lacking as well." Drugs in category D or X should never be taken during pregnancy, as studies have proven a definite risk to the fetus. If you have concerns about a particular drug or medication, ask your pharmacist about its pregnancy category. Make sure to let your physician know about any regular medications that you take so he can advise you about whether it is safe to continue.

Recreational Drugs

Drugs that we think of as "street drugs" are off-limits. Even occasionally using drugs like cocaine and marijuana are harmful to the conception process. Using these drugs places your baby-to-be at great risk for problems like growth retardation, mental problems, and addiction. If you have a problem with any type of drug, seek help in getting clean before attempting a pregnancy. Simply being pregnant won't make you stop using drugs.

Physical Readiness: Not Just for Women

People still seem to think of pregnancy and planning pregnancy as women's work. You've probably guessed by now that this is simply not true. Your partner will have a lot to do with how successful you are at becoming and staying healthy during pregnancy. In fact, today we know that men's health can and does affect the health of your baby-to-be.

Chemicals, drugs, and other toxins can affect sperm quality and quantity, and even alter the sperm on a chromosomal level. This is why it's extremely important that men take seriously the idea of preparing for pregnancy.

FACT

Male smoking can change sperm on a morphological level as well as change the seminal fluid that surrounds it; both of these can lead to decreased viability of that sperm. Smoking by the male also lowers the density and motility of the sperm. Some studies have also shown that sperm from male smokers may lead to birth defects and childhood cancers.

Exercise is an important part of any healthy lifestyle, especially for the man trying to achieve a pregnancy. There are a few things he needs to watch. Long-distance runners (those who run more than 100 miles a week) and cyclists who ride more than 50 miles per week may have lower sperm counts. The good news is that your sperm counts should return to normal if you temporarily alter your workout schedule.

By maintaining a healthy diet, a man also can help ensure his body is functioning at its prime. This enables all of his body systems to be in good working order. When his body is healthy, it makes healthy, high-quality sperm.

Unlike women, who are born with every egg they will ever have, a man begins to produce sperm when he starts puberty and will continue to do so his entire life. It takes about three months for sperm to mature, so the sperm that gets you pregnant today was created and raised in his body over the last three months. This means it was exposed to everything he was exposed to during that period. Your partner should think about making these healthier choices a few months before you attempt a pregnancy.

In addition to the simple physical standpoint of a healthy body, having your partner at your side as you make these lifestyle changes can make them easier to live with. In other words, a decision you make together is much easier to abide by than one you make alone. For example, if you decide it's time to add exercise to your life, what helps more? The partner lying on the couch while you go out and walk, or the partner who says, "Let's go together!"? It takes two to tango (and perform other forms of healthy living), so get on the ball and support each other in your new baby-friendly lifestyle.

Let's Talk about Sex

Sex is a natural, healthy, and intimate part of any marriage. Suddenly though, when undergoing infertility treatment, it can seem that your sex life is fair game for an entire office of complete strangers. You'll find yourself discussing your partner's sperm count, your cervical mucus, and your menstrual flow in great detail. In addition, being instructed to have sex by your doctor because you're ovulating can really kill the mood. Under those conditions, it's no wonder that many couples face issues with their sexual life.

Each clinic will have their own guidelines, and it is important to ask what their expectations are before you start treatment. Generally speaking, it is okay to have intercourse throughout your treatment time, but there may be times when you are asked to abstain. This is usually because they want your partner's sperm count to be optimal before having IUI or IVF. This period of abstinence is usually around two to three days, though it can be as long as five days before the procedure.

ESSENTIAL

One way to keep it fun is to not tell your partner when you are ovulating. Surprise him in a fun way instead! Not only does it keep things interesting, but it can help alleviate any performance anxiety on your partner's behalf.

Communication

Whether you choose to disclose the journey that you and your partner are about to embark on is a very personal decision, and whether you do so is up to you as a couple. Having this conversation before any awkward situations arise avoids any miscommunication and will make sure you're both on the same page.

Your Employer

On first thought, it may seem completely unnecessary to talk to your boss about such a personal problem. But over the course of the next several months, there may be many mornings where you need to come in to work late because of monitoring appointments, or take a last minute day off to fit in an IUI or IVF procedure. Keeping your boss in the loop (presuming you think he will be supportive of your need for flexibility) can make those last minute schedule changes a lot easier.

If you are concerned that your boss may hold this against you or not be supportive of what you are going through, don't feel obliged to tell. Your clinic may be able to provide you with a generic note stating that you are having a medical issue that requires frequent appointments.

Your Family and Friends

There are going to be times when you may need extra help over the course of the cycle. You may need a ride home after a procedure or some help food shopping if you are on bed rest. There are all sorts of little things that come up, and having family members or friends on board can ease some of those worries. Close friends and family can provide emotional support as well by giving you an extra shoulder to cry on or person to vent to—who isn't your partner.

You'd be amazed at how many people struggle with infertility or know someone who has. You might be surprised at some of the people who open up and share their stories with you.

Taking these steps to prepare for infertility treatment, and hopefully a pregnancy, will make it much easier on you in the long run. Getting healthy and staying healthy for a pregnancy can seem like an overwhelming task. The thoughtfulness that you put into readying your body is important, and will help ensure that you and your partner are at your peak readiness for your pregnancy and new baby.

CHAPTER 5

Selecting Your Doctor

Choosing your reproductive endocrinologist is a big decision. It's not just your relationship with her that's important, but the staff and how the clinic is run will also play a tremendous role in how you feel about cycling there. There are some important factors that you should consider before you decide on a clinic.

How to Find a Reproductive Endocrinologist (RE)

If it seems that an infertility evaluation is in your future, you will need to find a reproductive endocrinologist (RE)—a fancy term for a specialist who deals with the science of human reproduction. She has completed a general obstetrics and gynecology residency as well as additional specialty training in infertility.

Fellowship

During the reproductive endocrinology and infertility fellowship, the doctor is immersed in fertility issues nearly all of the time. Learning basic diagnostic testing for reproductive issues of both males and females is very important, and the doctor also begins to manage hormonal testing and medications for ovulation induction and IVF cycles. She learns how to perform advanced surgeries to diagnose and repair potential reproductive problems her patients may experience. Some of the things she learns are the IVF procedures and surgeries like hysteroscopies, laparoscopies, and other surgical techniques.

Board Certification

Finishing a fellowship allows a doctor to gain an enormous amount of knowledge about the field of reproductive endocrinology and infertility. She is not, however, certified in the field. To be board certified in reproductive endocrinology and infertility from the American Board of Obstetricians and Gynecologists (ABOG), doctors must pass both written and oral board examinations. This normally takes a couple of years post fellowship. Not all practitioners choose to obtain board certification for various reasons, so this is something you should ask about if you have a preference. Some insurance companies may even require that your RE be board certified for you to receive certain benefits.

Getting a Recommendation

So how exactly does one go about finding an RE? There are a couple of people you can ask for a recommendation. First, ask anybody you know who has gone through infertility treatment about her experiences at her clinic. Chances are she will be honest in her evaluation of the offices, including the negatives. This is important because you will want as much information as possible, and having it from a patient's perspective can be particularly helpful.

FACT

You can also check out the "Find a Member" page on the American Society for Reproductive Medicine's website, *www.asrm.org/FindAMember*. There are a variety of search fields, so you can search by name, zip code, and even type of service you are looking for.

If this isn't an option, try talking to your midwife or ob/gyn. They most likely have a number of relationships with infertility specialists and can provide you with a solid referral.

Making Sense of SART

Every year, fertility clinics that are members of the American Society for Reproductive Medicine (ASRM), the major professional organization representing fertility specialists, are required to submit their cycle statistics to an organization called the Society for Assisted Reproductive Technology, or SART, that works in close contact with the Centers for Disease Control, a branch of the federal government. Those statistics are available to the public and should be considered when selecting a clinic.

There are several important pieces of information you should consider when looking at a clinic's statistics. At the top of the report, you'll find a breakdown of the major diagnoses being treated at the clinic. For example, if you know that your partner has an issue with his sperm count, you'll want to find a clinic that has experience treating male factor infertility. If you want to further break down the statistics, there is a drop-down menu that will show you only the cycles done by the clinic that were due to male factor infertility. You can see the pregnancy rate, number of embryos transferred, and even the number of multiple pregnancies.

If you're not sure of what your diagnosis is yet, check out the total cycle statistics. What is the overall pregnancy rate for your age group? Were there many high order pregnancies (triplets or higher)? It may seem cute or even better to have triplets (because you're having several children all at once and are therefore "done"), but that is truly not a good sign. The goal of any clinic should be one healthy pregnancy. Being pregnant with high order multiples dramatically increases both a woman's and her babies' risk for complications.

ALERT

You can find the SART statistics online at *www.sart.org/find_frm.html*. Before making an appointment with a clinic, ensure that the clinic is a member of SART. It can be helpful to review their statistics as well.

Finally, down at the bottom of the page, there is information about the services offered at the clinic. Take a look and double check that what you need is available there.

How to Select a Clinic

Of course, the reputation and skill of the physician you'll be seeing is important to consider. However, there are several other equally important factors to consider as you make your decision.

Services Offered

During the course of your fertility testing and treatment, you may need access to several different types of tests or equipment. You will want to be sure that the fertility center you choose can easily accommodate these needs with a minimal hassle for you.

Do they have an in-house laboratory? You will have many tests that involve drawing blood or doing other types of lab work. Can all of these tests be performed on site? Will you or your partner have to go elsewhere for any of the tests or blood draws? What about semen analysis and urinalysis?

Ultrasound testing may also be a big part of what you need during your treatments. This type of testing is often used to monitor your ovaries and/or uterine lining during any given cycle. Does the fertility center have ultrasound equipment? Are the technicians using it certified to do the job they are doing? If they have weekend hours, is there a separate location for weekends?

You will also want to know what hospitals or surgical centers they are affiliated with for treatment and testing. Again, your insurance may play a part in all of this and dictate where you can receive treatment. Try to find a clinic that offers multiple hospital affiliations, if possible. You will also want to know what surgical procedures and tests they can perform in their clinic. For example, can they do in vitro fertilization in the clinic or is it done at another center?

The Staff

Once you've gotten a recommendation and reviewed the statistics, it's time to make an appointment. Pay attention to the process. Is the receptionist helpful? Pleasant? Is it easy to make an appointment? These are all important factors to consider as it is likely you will be in the office many times.

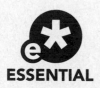

ESSENTIAL

Because the physicians are probably very busy, the nursing staff will be your main contact while you are undergoing a cycle. In most cases, they are incredible patient advocates and will work hard to make sure that your care goes smoothly. You must be able to trust them and have a good relationship with them. If you can't, you might want to consider finding a different clinic.

Is it easy to call and get a hold of someone to ask questions? Do they seem knowledgeable and easy to work with? Do they return your phone calls? Chances are you'll have plenty of medication and protocol questions as time goes by, and it is absolutely imperative that the staff be available or return your messages in a reasonable manner.

Is there someone to help you with insurance issues? Infertility coverage and financing is particularly nightmarish, and having someone help you sort through the details and straighten everything out is ideal.

The Physician

He might be an incredibly talented physician, but if he is not a good personality match, the relationship may be a disaster waiting to happen. You will be working closely with him over the coming months, and maybe even years, so it important that you and the physician have a good working relationship. Is the doctor sensitive to your concerns? Does he listen to your questions and answer them appropriately? Does he take the time to explain the process, and is he available for questions in between appointments? Trust is an absolute must in this business. If you can't trust your doctor, you should be seeing someone else.

The Office

Is the practice close to where you live or at least easy to get to? How is the parking? Once you start an IVF cycle, you will be in for monitoring every morning for close to two weeks. If you have a two- or three-hour commute to the office, think about how you'll feel making that drive on a daily basis. Are their monitoring hours convenient? Chances are that you'll still be going to work while cycling, so are you able to get from the clinic to your office in a timely fashion after your monitoring appointments? Is there a three-hour wait for monitoring each morning? Again, it may not be a big deal the first time it happens, but think about how you'll feel ten days in.

Preparing for Your First Visit

Getting a few things in order before your first visit with the doctor can help make the process much easier. Use this checklist to get you started.

- ❑ Call your insurance carrier.
- ❑ Determine your budget for treatment if it isn't covered by your insurance.

❑ Get copies of all of your previous testing or applicable medical records.

❑ Use the worksheet in Appendix A to list any questions/concerns before your appointment.

❑ Make sure you have the dates of your last few periods.

❑ Gather all of the materials you will need to bring with you and put in one place: medical records, period dates, basal body temperature charts (if applicable), and your list of questions.

Financial/Insurance Prep

It can be helpful to call your insurance carrier and determine the extent of your infertility coverage. If, for example, you have IVF coverage but only with three IUI cycles first (a common stipulation), this can be important information to share with the doctor so she doesn't automatically recommend IVF and cause challenges later as you realize that you are not covered for the treatment. Some insurance plans also require that one brand or another is the preferred one for the prescribed hormones. Again, having this information up front can prevent you from having to get a second prescription.

ALERT

Even if infertility treatment is not covered, your insurance may cover your initial testing and monitoring. Check with your carrier to see if they cover any of this lab work. If they do, they may require that you use a specific lab, so make sure that the office sends the blood to the appropriate place.

If you know going in that you will not have insurance coverage, this can impact your care also. IVF can be expensive, up to $15,000 a cycle, or even more if you are using donated eggs. In that situation, you'll want to think about what works best for your budget. Is it better to be more aggressive up front for a better chance at pregnancy? Or is it more feasible to use the least expensive options first while you save up for IVF? Having a basic understanding of your finances, and communicating that with your doctor, will make the process much smoother.

Your Medical History

If you've seen another specialist or had some preliminary tests done by your ob/gyn or midwife, request a copy of those records and test results. Taking a few minutes to reflect on your medical history can be helpful too; it's common for people to forget those details when sitting in a doctor's office. Gather the dates from your last few periods and your basal body temperature charts, if you're the one who has been doing the charting.

Use the worksheet in Appendix A to organize your thoughts and medical history. Writing your questions down before you walk into the office is really important. This way you'll be sure to get the answers you need by not forgetting the questions; a common phenomenon, especially if you get less than ideal news.

Knowing the Staff

In addition to your physician, there is a number of support staff whose job it is to make sure that your treatment goes as smoothly as possible. Getting to know who's who is an important part of navigating your way through infertility treatment.

The Nurses

The nurses coordinate your care throughout the office and tend to do a lot of the behind-the-scenes work. They make sure that you have the correct medication, coordinate the necessary procedures with the lab, work in the operating and recovery rooms, and review all lab results with the physician. The nurses will teach you how to do your injections and be available for questions throughout the day. They will also relay the physician's instructions to you.

The Lab Staff

Working in the lab are usually two types of specialists: embryologists and andrologists. Embryologists work primarily with the embryos by performing the fertilizations, assisting during egg retrievals and embryo transfers, and culturing the embryos throughout their development. They are responsible for overseeing your embryos through the entire process.

Andrologists manage the semen samples that are processed during semen analyses, IUIs, and sperm cryopreservation. They evaluate the quality of the sperm and relay that information to the physician.

Financial Associates

Your billing coordinator will help you deal with your insurance company and can help you find ways to navigate the complex policies. She ensures that the billing is done correctly and will often coordinate payment according to your facilities policy. She can also help answer questions about your coverage or help you find alternate funding sources through loans, medical financing programs, or even IVF specialty programs.

Genetic Counselor

Technology has advanced to a point where certain genetic diseases can be prevented through the use of a type of screening called preimplantation genetic diagnosis, or PGD. Additionally, most clinics screen couples to make sure that they aren't at risk for having a child with cystic fibrosis, Tay-Sachs, or other diseases based on their ethnic profile. The genetic counselor can be useful in helping a couple sort out their options and understand the results of their routine genetic screening.

FACT

PGD involves taking a biopsy from each of the embryos and analyzing it before the embryos are transferred back into the uterus. Some clinics are now even offering this procedure to help a couple have a child of a particular gender. Not all clinics offer this service, and you should ask up front if it is something you are interested in.

Not all clinics offer the services of a genetic counselor. Ask for a referral if yours doesn't, or check out *www.nsgc.org/resourcelink.cfm* to help you find someone locally.

Psychologist

Going through infertility treatment is draining, not just on your finances, but on your emotions and marriage as well. Most clinics require that you see a psychologist, often someone who has been specially trained in reproductive issues, before proceeding with IVF, using donated gametes, or both. These specialists are usually available throughout your entire cycle if you need them for additional support. Couples often feel that they're handling things "just fine," but it's important to take care of the little issues before they turn into big ones. If it's a requirement anyway, why not take advantage of the time you have with her and hash out some of your concerns?

Getting a Second Opinion

Sometimes the physician may recommend a treatment with which you strongly disagree. Perhaps you read something negative online or are not comfortable with the planned course of action (like using donated sperm or eggs). Maybe the doctor is recommending surgery and it doesn't feel quite right. If this happens, don't allow yourself to be pushed into something that you are not comfortable doing.

Don't ever hesitate to get a second opinion. The doctor or staff will not take it personally, and it is imperative that you are okay with your treatment plan.

If your second opinion backs up the first, you can use either physician for your treatment, depending on which office you felt more at ease with. If the two opinions vary or are dramatically different, you have a difficult decision to make. Be an informed consumer, and do as much research as possible.

ALERT

When researching infertility treatments, be wary of the advice given out on forums and discussion boards. The advice is probably from a layperson, based on her own personal experiences, and therefore may or may not be appropriate for you. Stick to professional organizations and medically reviewed sites for your research.

It also can't hurt to discuss the results of your second opinion with your first physician and see what she says. She may have some insight into why the other physician made the recommendations that he did and why she prefers her plan. After your research, you should have some idea of which plan you prefer. If all else fails, maybe a third opinion is in order. Do be aware, however, that "doctor shopping" and mixing and matching your care is a poor idea because it interrupts the continuity of your treatment.

CHAPTER 6

Show Me the Money

Nobody can say that infertility treatment is cheap. IVF cycles can easily run from $10,000 to $20,000 each, depending on your level of insurance coverage and the amount of medication you'll require. Quite often, even if you have insurance coverage, there are stipulations in your plan. You may need to complete a certain number of IUI cycles first, or only have three lifetime medication fills from your pharmacy. So, how do you make sense of it all and find the solution? Read on.

Health Insurance

There are no easy answers when it comes to insurance questions. Using your health insurance is the obvious answer to addressing the medical needs you are experiencing, but you may run into many problems when you submit your procedures for coverage.

Insurance Basics

Chances are, your health insurance is employer-based, meaning it is provided as a benefit through either your or your partner's employer. What your particular health insurance covers is not up to you; the employer determines your health insurance coverage. You may still have some choices, however.

It is very important that you let your employer know what coverage you want or need. Your employer may even be willing to add coverage for fertility treatments if they know that there is a demand, so this is worth looking into.

ALERT

Just because you work at the same company and have the same insurance carrier as another employee does not mean that you have the same coverage. Always be sure to read your policy before determining what your specific insurance covers.

Reading your policy is just the beginning. You are usually given a summary of benefits when you sign up for your health insurance. While this is a nice and tidy document, it is not your actual coverage list. Remember that it is your right to see your coverage in full detail. Ask your human resources department to see the contract they have with the health insurance carrier. You will want to read the sections that might particularly pertain to the treatment of infertility. Look at exclusions of coverage, as well as at limitations of coverage and of benefits. This might even include monetary limits on how much the insurance will spend on fertility treatments. If need be, ask for help with this document, as you need to be able to understand it in detail.

State Laws

A few states have a mandated insurance coverage for infertility treatment. However, that is not as promising as it seems. The majority of these states actually have a mandate that encourages employers to offer the services, but does not require coverage. This means that insurance companies in the state must *offer* a policy for purchase that covers infertility, but the laws don't require that the employer pay for the infertility services.

It probably goes without saying that you have a much better chance of getting coverage in states where coverage is mandatory. When a state mandates this kind of coverage, employers must provide insurance to cover the cost of infertility treatment in every premium, not as a separate expense.

Only fifteen states have passed legislation that requires some degree of infertility insurance coverage: Arkansas, Connecticut, California, Hawaii, Illinois, Louisiana, Maryland, Massachusetts, Montana, New Jersey, New York, Ohio, Rhode Island, Texas, and West Virginia. These laws vary widely according to the state in which you live. Check out *www.resolve.org/family-building-options/insurance_coverage/state-coverage.html* for more detailed information.

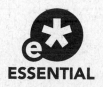

ESSENTIAL

Some infertility patients have gotten wise to the games insurance companies play. Be sure to have your care provider use diagnosis codes that do not reflect infertility as a diagnosis; rather, they should list the disease, like endometriosis or anovulation, instead of infertility secondary to anovulation. This is one way to get all or part of your treatments covered.

One loophole that many women can take advantage of states that you do not necessarily have to live in the state that has a mandate. If the company you work for is headquartered in a state that has mandatory infertility treatment coverage, even if it's not the state where you work and live, your health insurance is most likely provided through the state with the mandate. In this case, you'll be able to get the coverage too.

Even when your health insurance covers infertility testing or procedures, there are often exclusions or other problems with actually using the insurance. You may find that your insurance will only pay for certain procedures, like repairing your fallopian tubes, but not for in vitro fertilization.

Perhaps you are one of the lucky ones with great coverage, but you find that your insurance has a cap on it. This means that your plan will cover almost anything, but only up to a certain amount. After that, you're on your own.

Shared-Risk Programs

Shared-risk programs are designed to let you, funnily enough, "share the risk" of the costs with the fertility clinic. It usually only applies for IVF cycles, and not other forms of treatment or testing.

The typical way a shared-risk program works is that you pay, in full and up front, a certain reduced fee in exchange for a particular number of fertility procedures and cycles (usually three to five cycles). The promise is that, if you have not given birth by the end of the number of cycles initially agreed upon, all or a portion of your money is refunded to you. The amount of money refunded to you may depend on how many cycles you actually completed.

If you do get pregnant, carry that baby to term, and give birth to a live infant, even if after only one cycle, you do not get any of your money back. The fertility clinic keeps the rest of the money that you gave them, even though you only needed one cycle of treatment.

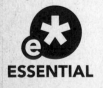

ESSENTIAL

You will usually have to meet certain criteria to enter a shared-risk program. You will probably have to be within a certain age. You may have to have a certain need for treatment, like IVF. And certain diagnoses may exclude you from participation in these programs.

In essence, you are banking on the fact that it is likely to take more than one cycle to get pregnant. If you do get pregnant on the first try, you have spent more money than you would have had you only paid for a single cycle. But if you do not get pregnant even after several cycles, you have lost no money, or at least considerably less money than you would have spent if not for the shared-risk program. Different clinics handle the particulars of the "refund" differently, so be sure you understand fully what your clinic's specific program entails.

QUESTION

How can I find a clinic that has a shared-risk program?
Not all fertility clinics offer shared-risk programs. If you are interested in this concept, ask around to find out what center closest to you participates in this type of program. Many couples actually travel great distances to take part in shared-risk cycles at fertility clinics that are far away from their homes.

You may also be expected to pay additional money for certain procedures. If you require intracytoplasmic sperm injection or the use of donor eggs, you may need to pay more money into your cycle. You may know this initially and have to pay right away, or your doctors may discover it as late as the day of your retrieval, in which case you'll be asked for the money then. Be sure to ask questions about these potential additional fees.

Special Programs

Another possible source of funding to help you pay for infertility testing and treatment are special programs. These may be run by universities or other groups doing studies, or even by drug companies. Programs like these sometimes pay for all or some of your treatments.

Medical Studies

Occasionally you may be able to find a university or other group doing a study that you can take part in. The researchers may be studying your particular diagnosis, or they might be studying a new medication or procedure that could help you achieve a pregnancy.

To find out if there are any of these types of programs near you, call your local medical school and ask to speak to someone who is conducting human research in reproductive endocrinology, or whatever subject your fertility issue would fall under, like urology. You may be referred to a general human studies center or you may be put through to a research nurse. You will likely be interviewed to see if you qualify for the study.

If you are lucky enough to find something that can help you foot at least part of your bill, you will likely have to give something in return. Typically, this is information in the way of data from your testing or procedures. This may mean that you have to have more blood work or additional procedures like ultrasounds so the researchers can get the data they need. You will also be asked to sign multiple waivers and releases.

Scholarships and Drug Companies

Another way to find some help paying for your medical expenses is to talk to drug companies. This can be a big help since the medications that are often required for the most advanced reproductive technologies can be a large portion of the bill. Several companies have programs set up to help you cover the costs of these medications.

Ask your fertility team if they are aware of any such programs. If they are, ask about how to get a hold of their contact person, normally a drug representative through a particular company. If your team is not aware of any such programs, have them ask. It certainly can't hurt, and it can only stand to benefit you and other patients in their practice.

These types of programs may have certain stipulations. For example, couples may have to meet certain income requirements—having a combined income under a certain amount—to qualify. It may also be diagnosis-related or even age-related. Follow up and see what you need to do to apply for such programs if you find them available to you and your partner.

Loans

Borrowing money may not seem like the ideal way to pay for treatments, but it is a way to make possible something that might otherwise not be.

The most obvious type of loan is a traditional bank loan, but this option is not available to everyone. It may depend on your credit rating, though there are some companies willing to overlook slightly negative credit ratings to help you out. Get a letter from your fertility practitioner that outlines how much money is required, what therapy is needed, and a breakdown of what each procedure will cost. He may also include any other information that he feels will help you get the loan. This will be a valuable document in your quest for a bank loan.

ESSENTIAL

Make sure to read the fine print very carefully before you take a loan. You don't want to be surprised by high interest rates or unreasonable payments that you can't afford. It might be helpful to discuss the terms with your accountant or financial planner beforehand.

You may even try asking other fertility patients what type of loan program they used. There are loan programs designed specifically for IVF patients. You should be sure to talk to previous customers to ensure you have some idea of how the service is for the program. Ask for references whenever possible. Your fertility center may even have a loan program available.

Another idea is to look into a second mortgage on your home. This is a fairly typical way to obtain extra cash for medical expenses, and it may actually have a lower interest rate than traditional loans.

Another option is to get a home equity loan that usually offers reasonable payment amounts on a monthly basis. You can also have a home equity line. The nice thing about a home equity line is that, once opened and partially paid off, you can always use it again and again. It can be used for multiples cycles over time.

Your Medication Coverage

Fertility medications can be quite expensive, sometimes up to fifty or sixty dollars *per vial* for your stimulation. If you're taking five or six vials a night, it can add up quickly. Coverage for your medication varies widely according to your insurance policy.

It can be helpful to call ahead of time to determine what, if anything, is covered. Sometimes a particular drug is on their preferred drug list, meaning it is the only one of its type that is covered. It's usually quite easy to clear this change with your doctor, though it may mean that you have to take more than one injection because of the way the medication is mixed.

Some people have tried to save money by skimping on their dosages. This is a bad idea. Each dose is specifically designed for you and is calculated to your body's response. But there are other ways to save money on purchasing medications.

You may be tempted to buy medication online or at a store other than a pharmacy that deals consumer to consumer. This may result in significant savings, but it comes with greatly increased risk. Be sure you have adequate safeguards in place to protect your interests financially, physically, and legally before you enter in to such a deal. Also bear in mind that medications have expiration dates. While they may not be harmful after the expiration date, they also may not work as well. You may find that you are left without medications or money or, even worse, that you are now ill from the medications that you purchased.

You may find your medications are less expensive if purchased from a pharmacy other than your local one. There are a multitude of pharmacies that do mail order or specialize in infertility medications, and these may be a better bargain for your buck.

ALERT

If you choose a mail order pharmacy, make sure you have an adequate supply of all of the medications you'll need over the course of your cycle. It can sometimes take a few days to get a delivery, and there are times when you need your medication right away; not having it can potentially screw up your cycle.

You may find that some fertility patients have medications left over from previous successful, or unsuccessful, cycles and are willing to sell these medications to you at a greatly reduced price. Your fertility clinic may even take part in this exchange of unused medications. Ask the program coordinator at your fertility clinic if she is aware of any such program locally.

Determining What You Can Afford

The difficult part about the financial decisions that accompany fertility treatments is that, of course, there is so much more involved than money. You have the basic need, urge, and right to become a family with children. You may feel like there are a lot of players making decisions for you about your own fertility—often without even knowing you. Be careful not do anything rash that would jeopardize your future, for you or your hopeful new family. Take the time to rationally think through each and every option. Do not take the first option that becomes available.

Shopping Around

One way to find the best bargain is the old-fashioned way—shop around. You may find that one fertility clinic offers you more in a cycle package than another does. Or you may find that overall costs are lower at a certain facility. Even better is when you find out that your insurance will cover some or all of your treatments or procedures if done at a certain location. Your fertility treatments cost too much financially and emotionally to leave any stone unturned.

One thing that many fertility patients are doing is being better consumers. You may be surprised to learn that not every doctor or clinic charges the same price for everything. Know up front what each cycle will cost and what that cost specifically includes. This means knowing what extra costs might creep up on you.

Price other local fertility centers, not just the first one you go to. You might find that what you thought was a great deal is really the opposite when you look at all the potential "extras" you may have to pay for. The middle of your cycle is not the time to find out that you need more tests or more medications or an additional medication. While these things can legitimately crop up unexpectedly, there should be very few surprises like this in the course of your treatment. You have a right to know about all of the potential medical and monetary expenses that may come your way.

Be Responsible

As always, be sure that you are financially responsible when dealing with loans. It is sad to say that many couples have gone into bankruptcy or gone through other monetary troubles in pursuing fertility treatments. Don't let the pursuit of a family jeopardize your ability to pay your bills.

If you are considering a shared-risk program, be sure it's a wise investment. Does your diagnosis make it seem more likely than average that you would get pregnant on an early attempt? It's a difficult question to answer, but it is also a tough gamble to make.

Budgeting and saving are ways to look into the future. They are also beneficial habits to get into, no matter which program you may ultimately decide on to help you finance your fertility treatments. Ask if your fertility clinic offers support in these areas. No matter what you decide to use to help you make the money to afford your fertility treatments, remember that you will be living with these decisions for a long time. Choose with guidance and wisdom. Seek help and support. In the end, do what works best for you to build your family.

CHAPTER 7

Diagnosing and Managing Male Factor Infertility

Evaluating your sperm is important because approximately 40 percent of couples seeking help for infertility are diagnosed with male factor infertility. If you have had a semen analysis (SA) that came back slightly abnormal, your doctor may recommend repeating the test. A severely low sperm count may require you to be evaluated by a urologist, a specialist in the urinary systems of both men and women, and in the reproductive health of men.

The Physical Exam

It may not be the most pleasant thing in the world, but having a physical exam by a urologist is an important part of the diagnostic process. By assessing your genitalia, the urologist can look for signs of low testosterone levels, varicoceles, or other structural issues which may be the cause of low sperm count. Having an idea of what to expect can make the process a little easier.

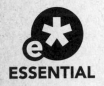

ESSENTIAL

If the RE requests a urology evaluation, ask for a referral. It is really important to consult someone who has experience working in the infertility field. The timing is absolutely crucial if surgery is required, and it can't be stressed enough that your urologist *MUST* understand what is required.

The urologist will ask you to remove your pants and underwear and put on a gown. He will then ask you to stand up and lift your gown.

He will look at and palpate (the medical word for touch) your penis and testicles to make sure that everything is structurally normal. He'll look to make sure that the urethral meatus (opening) is in the correct place, and that the testicles are firm and the appropriate size. He'll feel your testicles to make sure that the vas deferens and epididymis are present and feel normal.

Finally, the urologist may choose to do perform a digital rectal exam to assess the size of your prostate. To do this, the urologist will insert a gloved, lubricated finger into the rectum in order to feel the prostate. The exam will be very brief.

Semen Analysis

The semen analysis is the cornerstone of assessing male factor infertility because it gives your RE and the andrology staff the ability to look directly at your sperm. Are they normally formed and shaped? Are they moving appropriately? Are they alive? How many are there? The semen analysis can easily answer all of these questions.

You will need to abstain from ejaculation (both through sex and masturbation) for two to three days before you have a semen analysis. On the day of your appointment, you will need to ejaculate into a sterile container and give it to the laboratory staff. Production can be done through either masturbation or, if necessary, intercourse using a special condom kit that will collect the sperm.

ALERT

Don't use any lubricants if you choose to produce your sperm through intercourse, as many of them can negatively affect your sperm count. In most situations, canola oil is a good alternative, but definitely double check with the lab to make sure that this is okay.

Most centers have a collection room on site, but check with the staff to see if at-home production is an option if you are uncomfortable with producing in the office. There are usually some guidelines so you should ask about them when making the appointment. This way you can plan ahead in case you need to pick up a special container or need to schedule more time at home before the appointment.

"Producing on demand" can be stressful for many men. Performance anxiety and the fear that something might be wrong can be pretty potent when it comes to killing the mood. Anything you can do to help reduce this anxiety will help make the process easier. And hey, it may make it more fun, too!

Concentration

The concentration of the sperm sample is how many sperm cells are present per milliliter of semen. The concentration should be greater than 20 million sperm per milliliter. When the concentration is less than 20 million/ml, it's usually because of a lowered sperm count. The presence of a varicocele, stress, medication, or an illness can all cause a lowered sperm count.

Motility

The motility of a sample refers to how well and how many of the sperm cells are moving. Approximately 50 percent or more of the sperm cells should be moving appropriately. Sometimes you'll see sperm spinning in circles or simply shaking in place; that is not normal sperm movement. Low motility can be a sign of too long of a period of abstinence, the presence of anti-sperm antibodies, or other defect in spermatogenesis (process of making sperm).

Total Motile Count

This measures the total amount of normal, moving sperm cells in a given sample. It can be found by multiplying the volume of the semen produced by the concentration multiplied by the percent motility. You can also just ask the lab to give you the number, since they'll need to calculate it anyway for their records. Low counts indicate that either IUI or IVF may be necessary to optimize your chances for pregnancy.

Other Parameters

Besides the ones listed above, the lab technician will look at the following additional factors in your semen:

- **Volume of semen**—How much semen is produced? (Normally this is between 2–6 ml)
- **pH level**—Alkalinity or acidity, preferably a 7–8 on the pH scale
- **Sperm viscosity**—The thickness of the sample
- **Sperm liquefaction**—It should liquefy within about an hour
- **Sperm agglutination**—There should be no sperm sticking together

Other Sperm Testing

In addition to the standard tests performed during a semen analysis, there are other tests that can help the physician diagnose and treat your sperm issue.

Kruger Morphology

A Kruger strict morphology count measures the percentage of normally shaped sperm. A sperm cell has three parts: head, midpiece, and tail. Each sperm cell must be absolutely perfect in order to be counted as normal. Even a slight deviation requires that it be assigned to the abnormal category.

The andrologist who performs the Kruger analysis will look at a set number of sperm cells in the specimen; usually around two hundred. When doing the analysis, she will actually measure five unique components in each sperm.

FACT

Unlike a semen analysis, which can change from ejaculate to ejaculate, the results of a Kruger morphology test are relatively stable. There shouldn't be wide variations in your results in the short term.

Each lab will have its own set of standards; some use 4 percent normal sperm as their cutoff value, others will use 14 percent normal. Make sure to speak with your lab or other clinical staff member about their standards. With a very low value, IVF with ICSI is usually indicated.

Sperm Chromatin Structure Assay (SCSA)

The purpose of this test is to look at the actual DNA within the sperm cells. DNA is the genetic material found in the chromosomes that, if abnormal, can affect the ability of the sperm to penetrate and fertilize an egg. This test can be quite expensive and is not usually covered by your insurance.

Anti-Sperm Antibody Test

Problems with your immune system, and the immune system of your partner, are also part of the conception picture. Your semen may be tested for anti-sperm antibodies (ASA). You may need to have your blood tested also. The presence of ASA is much more common in infertile men (about 10 percent of infertile men versus 1 percent of fertile men and 0.5 percent of infertile women). The most likely cause is some type of damage or injury that has broken the blood-testes barrier that protects the sperm from the body's immune system. This may be something as invasive as a vasectomy (and reversal), hernia repair, or other testicular surgeries, to something as simple as a twisted testicle. Typically, using intrauterine insemination or even in vitro fertilization can help when ASA has been diagnosed.

Hormone Testing

If the semen analysis or other semen screening tests came back abnormal, the next step is to determine the cause and how to fix it. Much of sperm production is governed by the level of testosterone in your body, though many other hormones, like the thyroid hormones, prolactin, and testosterone all play a role as well. These can all be measured with a simple blood test.

Testosterone

Testosterone is essential to the making of sperm. When the testosterone levels are lower than expected, sperm production is negatively affected. One of the causes of decreased testosterone is hypogonadism. This generic catch-all term encompasses several causes of lowered testosterone production, including testicular disorders; problems with the hormonal regulating system in the pituitary or hypothalamus glands in the brain; congenital defects; and damage to the testicles or hormonal control system either by surgery, trauma, cancer, or lesions.

Thyroid disease

Studies have shown that both hypothyroidism (too little thyroid hormone) and hyperthyroidism (too much thyroid hormone) can affect a man's ability to maintain an erection and ejaculate, and can even lower his sex drive. Premature ejaculation is a common complaint as well.

ALERT

Thyroid issues can be a significant cause of infertility in men. Many practitioners who are not fertility specialists may not be aware of the significant problems caused by slight alterations in thyroid function. Thyroid expert Mary Shomon can help you with thyroid basics at *http://thyroid.about.com.*

While complaints with your sexual life can be difficult to talk about, it is important to mention them to your infertility specialist or your urologist because the embarrassing symptoms may actually be the result of a physical problem that is easily diagnosed and treated.

Prolactin

Hyperprolactinemia is a condition in which the pituitary gland produces too much prolactin. If a man's body produces too much prolactin, he can suffer from infertility. Too much prolactin can lead to lowered levels of follicle stimulating hormone (FSH) and luteinizing hormone (LH), which will alter sperm production. It can be caused by many things, such as blood pressure and other medications, pituitary tumors, or hypothyroidism (in which the pituitary does not release the proper amounts of hormones, resulting in excess prolactin being produced).

Sufferers may find that they have a loss of interest in sex, or a lower libido. Headaches or vision disturbances are also symptoms. About 30 percent of all cases of hyperprolactinemia are of an undetermined cause.

Genetics

Genetics sometimes play a role in contributing to azoospermia; one study suggested that approximately 6 percent of infertile men had an underlying genetic disorder. While the statistics seem low, it may be worth investigating this route if no other reason for the low sperm count can be found. Simply having the information can help you and the doctor find the best treatment available to prevent passing the defective gene down to future generations. It can also be beneficial to know that the infertility is a result of a genetic defect, and not a preventable behavior, like drug use.

Karyotype

The normal male karyotype is 46XY, meaning that he has one X chromosome and one Y chromosome. One relatively common deviation, occurring in about one in five hundred live male births, is XXY, called Klinefelter's syndrome. Men with this disease typically have small firm testes, obesity, decreased intelligence, and decreased development of secondary sex characteristics. Tests will show that FSH levels are elevated, and estradiol and testosterone levels are either normal or increased. Men with Klinefelter's syndrome don't usually produce much, if any, sperm.

Y Chromosome Microdeletion

The genes for spermatogenesis (the process of making sperm) are found on particular sections of the Y chromosome. If the information available in one or more of these sections is missing, the male will be normal by all appearances but may or may not produce viable sperm, depending on the location of the microdeletion. It is important to know that this genetic abnormality can be passed down to male children, so evaluation is definitely warranted. This can be tested for in a simple blood test. This test is not included in the standard karyotype test, so check with your doctor to see if he is ordering this one as well.

Overcoming Male Factor

There are many available interventions to help you increase your sperm count or even harvest a few healthy sperm cells for IVF. These techniques are only useful when there are some sperm cells to work with; after all, it only takes one sperm cell to fertilize an egg. Having at least as many sperm as there are eggs gives you a good chance of having some of the eggs fertilize. If you don't produce any sperm at all, you may need to discuss the option of using donated sperm.

Surgery

Surgery is a very aggressive form of treatment and should not be considered lightly. When considering urological surgery, be sure to also consult your fertility physician. Many times, the procedure will be done right before your egg retrieval, so the timing can get a little tricky.

ALERT

Using fresh sperm is ideal when going through IVF. This means that you (and your urologist) may only have a day or two's notice before surgery must be planned. This can of course be inconvenient, but your urologist must understand that he may need to rearrange his schedule at the last minute because your surgery cannot wait.

Using a physician your urologist is accustomed to working with can make the process smoother. Of course, if you are not comfortable with his recommendation, you have other alternatives. Your urologist can do the procedure at his convenience and have the tissue couriered to your facility to be frozen, though this is less than ideal.

There are a few different types of surgery:

- **Varicocele removal:** Removing a varicocele can help restore fertility. This should be done and your semen analysis reevaluated prior to starting treatment.
- **Microsurgical Epididymal Sperm Aspiration, or MESA:** The surgeon will make a small incision in the scrotum and aspirate sperm cells from the epididymis on each testicle. This procedure typically has a good success rate for sperm retrieval, but can be expensive and the recovery can be longer.
- **Percutaneous Epididymal Sperm Aspiration, or PESA:** The surgeon will use a needle to puncture the epididymis in several places and attempt to aspirate sperm cells through the needle. The procedure is typically done in the office, but has a higher chance of injuring the testicular structures because it is considered a blind procedure, i.e., the surgeon does not make an incision and is not able to directly visualize where the needle is being placed.
- **Testicular Epididymal Sperm Extraction, or TESE:** One or both of the testicles is opened up and samples of the tissue are removed. Those samples are then examined under the microscope for the presence of sperm cells. Again, this is an open procedure and recovery can be tough.

The last three procedures are usually only indicated in cases of obstructive azoospermia, where the sperm cells are being produced but are prevented from being ejaculated because of a blockage in the tubes connecting the testicles to the urethra. TESE is sometimes called for in cases where sperm production is uncertain. You should definitely have a detailed conversation with your urologist and even think about getting a second opinion before consenting to surgery.

Electroejaculation

In men who have difficulty ejaculating, the urologist can use special techniques to assist him. Usually done under anesthesia, a small probe is inserted into the rectum and small jolts of electricity are applied to the prostate to help stimulate ejaculation. The sperm is then collected and analyzed in the lab.

If retrograde ejaculation is the problem, a catheter is also inserted through the penis and into the bladder in order to drain the urine. The fluid is also analyzed and any found sperm cells are washed.

Recovery is generally pretty simple and just a matter of safely waking up from the anesthesia. You may have some slight discomfort that should be temporary and resolve fairly quickly.

Medications

It may surprise you to learn that there are infertility medications for men. In a few instances of male infertility, medications can be beneficial. Only your doctor can determine when or if medication therapy is the right treatment for you.

You may be prescribed a form of hormone replacement if you suffer from a pituitary disorder or some other problem that alters your body's production of LH or FSH. This is usually done in the form of a supplemental hormone or something to help the body boost the production of the LH and FSH on its own. Examples of these medications are Pergonal, Novarel, Pregnyl, Profasi, and Repronex. Even Clomid is sometimes used because it also indirectly raises the FSH level.

Producing enough testosterone may also be a problem for some men, even with the above therapies. There are also supplements available for this. Testosterone can be taken via deep intramuscular injection, implant, or through a testosterone patch. Testosterone is not an oral medication, as it is not broken down correctly if taken orally. Replacement testosterone gels have also recently become available.

Reversing a Vasectomy

Vasectomies are surgeries done to make a man infertile, and are used as a permanent, and very effective, form of birth control. For a variety of reasons, you and your partner may be choosing to try to have children after you have had a vasectomy.

In a vasectomy, the vas deferens is severed to prevent sperm from traveling out of the urethra. This can be done as an office procedure or as an outpatient surgery, as it's a minor procedure. After about twelve ejaculations postsurgery, the physician will perform a sperm count to see if the surgery was a success.

ALERT

While a vasectomy can be reversed, the procedure is much more invasive. If there is any chance that you will want additional children, it is recommended that you freeze a few vials of sperm prior to your vasectomy. Thawing a frozen vial is much easier than going through surgery again if you change your mind.

There are a few options available to regain fertility after a vasectomy. Microsurgery to try to repair the vas deferens is one option. The goal of the microsurgery is to make the vas deferens patent again so that sperm can flow freely through the reproductive tract for ejaculation. If successful, the surgery to reverse the vasectomy will be all that is needed, and normal sexuality activity and attempts to conceive can go forward without much other intervention. Though the success rates of vasectomy reversals vary widely, the biggest factor is usually the length of time between the surgery and the repair.

There are also techniques to remove sperm directly from the testicles. This can be done through fine needle aspiration and the removal of testicular tissue. The problem with these methods is that they result in a limited number of sperm and require that the woman go through the in vitro fertilization process.

CHAPTER 8

Diagnosing Female Factor Infertility

Diagnosing female factor infertility is a complex process. There are a multitude of tests that your doctor will use to investigate the cause of your infertility. Most of your early testing will consist of simple blood tests and ultrasounds. Even those simple tests can yield a tremendous amount of information. In addition, your doctor will need to screen you for other hormonal and infectious diseases to ensure that you are healthy enough to conceive.

Testing Ovarian Reserve

Because a woman is born with all of the eggs she'll ever need, her eggs do age. Women do not ever make new eggs; as she ages, so do her eggs. This ovarian aging process is different for everyone; some women go through menopause at age fifty, others start the ovarian aging process as young as their twenties. Ovarian reserve refers to the number of quality eggs you have remaining in your ovaries.

Day Three Testing

This is the gold standard for testing ovarian reserve, and will probably be one of the first tests your doctor requests. It's very simple: just a blood test on the second, third, or fourth day of your period. The test will be for your estradiol (E2) and FSH levels. An elevated level of either of these hormones in the beginning of your period indicates that your ovarian reserve is declining.

FSH is the hormone produced by the pituitary gland, which recruits an egg follicle for development and maturity. As the number of eggs in your ovaries decreases, it takes more and more FSH to recruit an egg. A normal FSH level is one that is below 10 mIU/ml.

Estradiol is also measured as an indicator of ovarian reserve. Women who are in ovarian failure tend to have much shorter cycles, meaning that they will be ready to ovulate much earlier in their cycle. This causes the E2 level to be higher in the beginning of the cycle because a follicle is already maturing. The elevated E2 opposes the FSH level, keeping it low. Without seeing that the E2 level is high, the FSH may be mistakenly seen as normal. A normal E2 is one that is below 80mIU/ml.

Anti-Müllerian Hormone

Anti-Müllerian Hormone (AMH) is a relatively new blood test that is also being used to assess ovarian reserve. AMH, which is also known as Müllerian Inhibiting Substance or MIS, is produced by the egg follicles on the ovary. It is not affected by taking the birth control pill or the point you are in your cycle, the way FSH is. The fewer follicles you have, the lower your AMH will be.

The normal values for AMH are 0.7ng/ml to 3.5ng/ml. If your AMH is below 0.7ng/ml, it suggests that your ovarian reserve is low and that your response to the infertility meds will probably not be substantial.

FACT

AMH isn't just used to diagnose diminished ovarian reserve. If your AMH is elevated above 3.5ng/ml, it can possibly indicate PCOS. PCOS is characterized by lots of small egg follicles on the ovaries, which is why it would make sense to see high levels of AMH.

Antral Follicle Count

Each month, your body produces multiple egg follicles, not just one, as is commonly thought. Most of them are resting, or antral, follicles. The dominant follicle is the one that will go on to contain a mature egg inside and eventually ovulate. In the beginning of the month, your doctor may perform a transvaginal ultrasound to look at your ovaries and count the number of resting follicles you have. The more resting follicles you have, the better your ovarian reserve is presumed to be. These resting follicles are much smaller, usually around 2mm to 8mm, than the dominant follicle. The dominant follicle will grow to about 17mm or as big as 25mm at the time of ovulation.

Testing Other Hormones

Your hormone levels play a huge part in the overall makeup of your general fertility. Some of the easiest tests that determine fertility issues will be done with blood draws to check the levels of certain hormones in your body. Your team of fertility experts will then review this information and discuss with you what the lab work means and how to proceed from this point.

Prolactin

Prolactin is a hormone, produced by the pituitary gland, which is involved in lactation. High levels of prolactin can prevent FSH and LH from being secreted, which in turn suppresses ovulation. Testing your prolactin level can help detect a relatively easy-to-fix hormonal problem. Depending on your lab's specifications, a normal prolactin level is between 3ng/ml and 25ng/ml. There are other things that can temporarily increase your prolactin: sex, breast stimulation, and even eating. If your initial level comes back a little high, ask about retesting on a day when you can avoid all of those other factors.

The Thyroid Hormones

The hormonal systems in your body work intricately together to move toward pregnancy, so your thyroid plays a large part in your fertility. If you are experiencing fertility problems or you are having difficulty in conceiving, your practitioner may suggest that you have your thyroid hormones checked, as altered levels may increase the likelihood of infertility.

By checking your thyroid stimulating hormone (TSH) levels and other thyroid hormones, you can get an overall picture of your thyroid's functioning. If there are indeed problems with your thyroid, a simple medication to help regulate these hormones can have a tremendous effect on your ability to get pregnant.

Progesterone

Your progesterone levels may be checked to determine if your body is producing enough progesterone to sustain a pregnancy. Progesterone begins to rise midcycle, peaking just before menstruation would begin. If a pregnancy has occurred, the progesterone continues to rise. If you did not conceive, your progesterone levels fall, indicating a start to your menstrual flow.

ESSENTIAL

Some of the stimulant medications that you will take can also suppress your natural production of progesterone. Your doctor will likely prescribe additional progesterone supplementation that you will take during the luteal phase of your cycle to ensure that you have enough progesterone to support an early pregnancy.

Sometimes your progesterone falls even when you are pregnant, and a pregnancy loss occurs. Doctors and researchers do not yet know if the progesterone falls because the pregnancy is lost, or if a drop in progesterone actually causes the pregnancy to be lost. Taking progesterone supplements may help, and is also designed to help sustain a pregnancy in case it is the drop in progesterone that causes the loss.

Clomid Challenge Test (CCCT)

The Clomid Challenge Test (CCCT) is used to help determine ovarian reserve, or how well your ovaries function. Your follicle stimulating hormone (FSH) and estradiol (E2) levels will be tested on day three. You will then be prescribed Clomid (Clomiphene Citrate, 100 mg) from cycle days five through nine. Your FSH and E2 levels will again be checked on day ten. Both day three lab values (FSH and E2) and your day ten lab values should be within normal limits to be considered normal. If your day ten FSH levels are higher than 10 mIU/ml, you are said to have diminished ovarian reserve. This test is commonly used in women over thirty-five, or if your practitioner suspects that you may have premature ovarian failure.

Infectious Disease Testing

In addition to your hormonal testing, your physician will need to screen both you and your partner for some of the basic infectious diseases. This is partly for your protection, but also for the protection of the clinic. Depending on your clinic's policy, HIV, hepatitis B and C, and syphilis are common diseases screened for. They may also check to see if you've been exposed to chlamydia or gonorrhea through cervical cultures. Positive results don't mean that you won't be able to be treated, but may actually give a clue about the cause of your infertility. Many of the sexually transmitted infections can cause scarring in the reproductive tract and will need to be treated before conception occurs.

Because the clinic is either inseminating sperm or transferring embryos created with your partner's sperm into your uterus, they need to be absolutely certain that they are not transmitting any infectious diseases, including HIV and hepatitis. It is not uncommon for people to be unaware that they have hepatitis or even HIV, and for that reason everybody must be screened.

Finally, the FDA and Department of Health regulate what occurs in the laboratory and, they have strict requirements about how the sperm, egg cells, and embryos are handled and stored. If a patient has HIV or hepatitis, her body fluids must be quarantined away from the rest of the stored embryos and sperm/egg cells. This is to protect unaffected cells from being accidently infected and subsequently infecting the woman after insemination or embryo transfer.

ESSENTIAL

Your clinic may have other requirements that must be completed prior to your initiating treatment, depending on their policy. A letter of medical clearance from a doctor managing a particular health issue, up-to-date Pap smear, and recent mammogram are all common requirements.

Thrombophilia Panel

Not every practice will require a full thrombophilia screen before cycling, but some may. A thrombophilia panel looks at all of the different clotting factors involved in forming a blood clot. If the test reveals that you have a thrombophilia, it means that your body has a tendency to form clots easily. Most people with a thrombophilia don't even know they have it unless they've already had a blood clot, or thrombus.

One of the dangers of thrombophilia is a blood clot forming in the body, then breaking off and traveling to the heart, lungs, or brain where it can block blood flow. If that happens, a stroke or heart attack can occur. Having a clot while pregnant can be especially worrisome because there is a risk of developing a blood clot in the placenta or umbilical cord, which can block blood flow to the fetus. This can cause a number of problems, including fetal demise, premature delivery, recurrent pregnancy loss, and preeclampsia.

There are two types of thrombophilias: inherited or acquired.

Inherited Thrombophilias

Inherited thrombophilias are a result of a genetic defect that is passed down from your parents, and are a lot more common than acquired thrombophilias. The most common inherited thrombophilia is a mutation in the factor V Leiden gene. This gene mutation is most frequently found in Caucasians, at around 5 percent, and is rather rare in the Hispanic and African American populations.

The clotting process is very complex. In fact, there are many proteins and factors that must all be functioning properly in order for a clot to form. If there are either excessive or deficient levels of any of these components, your ability to clot is affected. When checking for inherited thrombophilias, your doctor will also look at the levels of these factors, specifically protein S, protein C, and antithrombin III. If any of these three proteins are abnormally low, you are at a higher risk for forming blood clots.

Acquired Thrombophilias

Acquired thrombophilias occur most commonly when antibodies are produced in the body that stimulate clotting. Again, any abnormal tendency toward blood clotting can cause a clot, or thrombus, to form in the venous system when it's not appropriate. Pieces of a clot can break off and travel through the circulatory system, where it can cause catastrophic consequences if lodged in the heart, lungs, or brain.

These antibodies typically form after some sort of trauma, like surgery, an injury, or certain other medical conditions.

Treating a Thrombophilia

If your doctor finds an abnormality in your thrombophilia testing, treatment varies according to the particular protein that is affected. Certain dysfunctions require no treatment at all. Sometimes a medication called Metanx, which is basically a combination of the B vitamins and additional folic acid, is recommended. You will take one of these pills every day while trying to conceive, during pregnancy, and even after delivery.

The other medication your doctor might prescribe is a blood thinner, which will prevent blood clots from forming. An injectable medication called Lovenox is the usual choice, which is normally taken once you have a positive pregnancy test. Some practitioners may have you start taking the Lovenox right after your embryo transfer, if you are being treated with IVF. Depending on the particular thrombophilia you have, you may need to continue taking the Lovenox throughout your entire pregnancy, or you may be able to stop it once you reach a certain point. That decision is up to your obstetrician. It can be helpful to have copies of your thrombophilia testing to show to your doctor.

ALERT

Metanx can be quite expensive and may or may not be covered by your insurance carrier. If it is not, check with your physician to see if there are alternatives. In some cases you can take over-the-counter supplements of folic acid and vitamin B in addition to your prenatal vitamin.

Genetics

Just as your partner may have needed to have some genetic testing, you may need to as well. If your partner was found to be a carrier of a genetic disease, like cystic fibrosis or Tay-Sachs disease, you will need to be tested to make sure that you don't carry the gene as well. Depending on how the disease is transmitted, you may risk having a child who suffers from the disease if both of you are carriers for the disease. Your doctor may recommend testing for other genetic diseases depending on your family history and, because certain diseases are more prevalent in certain populations, your ethnicity.

Karyotype

The karyotype of a normal female is 46XX. This means that she has a total of forty-six chromosomes, including the two X chromosomes that determine that she is female. If chromosomes do not divide properly during early development, this could lead to too few or too many body chromosomes. Most of these conditions are not compatible with life and would lead to death of the fetus in utero. However, there are a few conditions that could survive the pregnancy; Down's syndrome is one example. This condition, which is also called Trisomy 21, means that the child has three copies of the twenty-first chromosome.

A female child can also have an abnormal number of X chromosomes. Having only one X chromosome is found in a condition called Monosomy X, or Turner's syndrome. Many of these children die before birth, but those who survive do not go through puberty or develop the typical female sex characteristics. Women with Turner's syndrome are usually unable to have children and are considerably smaller in stature.

If a female child has three X chromosomes, her condition is called Trisomy X. Women with this condition are usually perfectly healthy. In fact, without seeing the karyotype results, you would never even know that they have this condition.

Fragile X

Each chromosome is made up of many, many genes. These genes are made up of molecules of DNA denoted by their initial: A, C, G, and T. It is the different combinations of those DNA molecules that make up each of the genes on the chromosome. Fragile X syndrome is a disease where one tip of the X chromosomes has an abnormally high number of a particular group of DNA segments that makes the end of the X chromosome unstable, or fragile.

Fragile X can affect both males and females, since both genders carry an X chromosome. Affected individuals often have intellectual disabilities and some degree of mental retardation. There are also a range of physical effects, including mitral valve prolapse, joint disorders, and a long face with a prominent chin and large ears. Because this disease is relatively common—approximately one in 4,000 to 6,000 females and one in 3,600 males are diagnosed with Fragile X—some physicians opt to routinely test all of their patients to see if they are carriers for the disease.

Other Tests

In addition to the usual diagnostic tests, your doctor may want to conduct other exams to determine if your body is ready to become pregnant.

Pregnancy can be a strain on the body, and the doctor will want to make sure that you are in top health before your pregnancy.

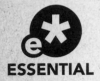

ESSENTIAL

Many experts now recommend a preconception appointment with your doctor to discuss your health and what to expect from a pregnancy. It's also a good way to select your ob/gyn and make sure that you like her before you discover that you are pregnant and are now in a rush to find a doctor you like.

Of course, pregnancy just happens in many situations without the benefit of preconception counseling. But if you are going to be spending a lot of time, money, and effort trying to get pregnant, why not make sure everything goes as smoothly as possible?

Blood Chemistry and Complete Blood Count

These two tests give a general picture of your overall health. The blood count can help diagnose anemia or other blood conditions. It's also really important to have a baseline blood count before your egg retrieval or surgery, if that is in your plan. Changes in the blood count can help diagnose a bleeding problem after surgery. Having a baseline is crucial in case of a problem during surgery. It's not something that most people like to think about, but it's an important precaution that your surgeon should take. He'll also want to check your blood type for the same reason.

Testing your blood chemistry can give the doctor an indication of how well your liver and kidneys are working. Certain medications can adversely affect their functioning, and the doctor will want to make sure that everything is okay before beginning treatment. This is particularly important before starting a medication like Metformin (Glucophage) for PCOS. Both of these may need to be periodically repeated during your treatment.

Vaccine Titers

Certain common diseases can negatively affect a pregnancy. Chicken pox and rubella in particular can cause serious birth defects and complications.

These diseases, however, are easily vaccinated against. Chances are you've had the immunizations in the past, but sometimes your immune response can decrease. Luckily though, you can easily check to see if you are still immune to either of those conditions. If you are, you will not need any further immunizations; if the blood test shows that you are not, you may need to retake the vaccination and then wait a period of time before you can become pregnant.

It may be tempting to skip the vaccination if the test shows that you need it, but given the severity of the potential complications, why take the chance?

CHAPTER 9

Diagnostic Procedures

In addition to the standard bloodwork and sonography, there are lots of other procedures that can give your reproductive endocrinologist (RE) information about the potential causes of your infertility. Surgery, specialized ultrasounds and x-rays, and post coital testing all provide important diagnostic clues. These procedures are not appropriate for everyone, but your doctor will decide what's best for you, given your whole clinical picture.

Hysterosalpingogram (HSG)

If your doctor suspects that you might have tubal factor, he'll want to check the status of your Fallopian tubes. This test is usually performed at a radiology center. The radiologist will insert a speculum into your vagina so that she can visualize your cervix. He will pass a special catheter into the uterus and inject a radio-opaque dye. The dye will fill the uterus, should pass through the Fallopian tubes, and will then spill out into the abdominal cavity. An x-ray will be taken to see if the dye is able to move through the tubes.

Preparation for Your HSG

Having an HSG requires a little more preparation than your standard x-ray or ultrasound. Appointments are only made on certain days of your cycle, usually day six through day eleven or twelve, to ensure that you are not pregnant, as the dye can disrupt the pregnancy. Your doctor may recommend that you take antibiotics before the test because you are at risk for infection whenever anything is introduced into the uterus. Preprocedure antibiotics can help minimize that risk, though you should still report any signs of infection—fever, severe cramping, or unusual vaginal discharge.

ALERT

Make sure to mention to both your doctor and the radiologist if you are allergic to any food or medications. Some people can have a severe allergic reaction to the dye. An even seemingly unrelated allergy may provide a clue as to whether you'll be able to tolerate the dye.

The facility will probably suggest that you take an anti-inflammatory two hours before the procedure to help minimize cramping. Most women do experience some discomfort, so make sure to take the recommended dose at the right time.

The Results

After the x-ray is developed, the radiologist and your doctor will both analyze the films to see exactly where the dye goes. Does it go all the way through the tube and spill into the abdominal cavity? If spillage is noted in the abdominal cavity, it is presumed that the Fallopian tube is open. If it does not, this indicates that one or both tubes are blocked.

An HSG can also look for the presence of a hydrosalpinx, which is a collection of clear fluid in the tube. A hydrosalpinx has a characteristic "sausage" look on the x-ray or ultrasound. Usually caused by an untreated chlamydia or gonorrhea infection, a hydrosalpinx often blocks the tube, causing infertility.

Post Coital Testing

A post coital test (PCT) is a check of your cervical mucous after you and your partner have had sexual intercourse. The test is usually done around the time of ovulation, so your doctor may ask you to come to the office periodically for monitoring to determine when you are actually about to ovulate. You can also usually use an ovulation predictor kit at home to test for your ovulation. Using a kit may not be appropriate for you, especially if you've had difficulty interpreting the test results in the past, or if you have PCOS. Of course you need to follow your doctor's instructions, but generally once you see the positive result, you will call the office and inform the staff. They will then help you schedule your PCT.

Preparing for Your PCT

You will be asked to come in to the office for the test within 4–10 hours after you and your partner have had sex. It is important that you follow these directions carefully.

The actual test is just like having a regular pap smear. Your care provider or a nurse practitioner will insert a speculum into your vagina and take a sampling of your cervical mucous while you are lying down on the exam table. This mucous will then be analyzed for several factors using a microscope. They will be looking at the amount and color of your cervical mucous, the amount of live sperm, the absence of other cells, and its ability to stretch. They will also most likely test your cervical mucous for indications of infection.

Your Results

Your cervical mucus changes in color and consistency once you've ovulated. Sperm cells also don't typically survive well in postovulatory mucus, so the results will be inaccurate if the test is done at the wrong time in your cycle.

This test can tell your care provider if your partner's sperm can penetrate the cervical mucous and survive. Abnormal results to this test may indicate a problem with your production of cervical mucous or with your partner's sperm viability.

FACT

Sometimes a PCT can be used as a preliminary diagnostic test for male factor infertility. If there are many sperm cells in the mucus, then male factor infertility is unlikely. On the other hand, if there are no sperm cells observed in the mucus, it can indicate the need for further testing.

Problems with the cervical mucous can be caused by a number of factors including medications, poor timing, an infection, or even cervical injury from prior procedures like cryosurgery or Loop Electrosurgical Excision Procedure (LEEP), a procedure in which a small loop is used to pass electrical current through to burn the cells off the cervix. Make sure to disclose any relevant medical history to the person doing your post coital exam. It is important that she has all of the necessary information when analyzing your results.

Endometrial Biopsy

Having a healthy endometrium is an important part of conception; otherwise, implantation could not occur. If you are having difficulty becoming pregnant when all other testing is within the normal range and you are responding well to the hormonal stimulation, the doctor may recommend that a biopsy of your uterine lining should be done. Some clinics may still require this as a prerequisite for anyone about to undergo IVF, even though current research no longer supports the efficacy of this practice.

An endometrial biopsy is used to define the quality of your uterine lining. This test will tell your doctor if your uterine lining is capable of sustaining a pregnancy. If there are problems found, you may need treatment with hormones to supplement your uterine lining.

ALERT

Do not perform this test if you could be pregnant, as it could disrupt your pregnancy. If there is any possibility that you could be pregnant, make sure to let you physician know beforehand.

This test is an in-office procedure and can be done by your doctor or the nurse practitioner. It is typically done one to three days before you expect your period. During this time your uterus should be thick and full of nutrients designed to sustain a pregnancy.

What to Expect During an Endometrial Biopsy

You will lie back on an exam table and a speculum will be inserted into your vagina. The doctor will look at and clean your cervix with a mild solution. A small catheter is then placed inside the uterus and moved back and forth, gathering a sample of the uterine lining. The doctor will likely want to take samples from a few locations within the uterus. The tissue is collected in a special container and sent to a lab for analysis. The procedure only takes a few minutes and does not require anesthesia; mild cramping is usually the only side effect. Check with your doctor, but it is probably okay if you take a mild pain killer like Tylenol two hours before your procedure to minimize the cramping.

Your Results

The technicians in the lab will check a few things. First, they will want to make sure that the endometrial tissue they received is in phase and appropriately developed. Remember that the endometrium is a tissue that responds to hormonal stimulation and therefore changes over the course of your menstrual cycle. The endometrial tissue should be sufficiently developed according to where you are in your cycle.

The lab techs will also check that special proteins called integrins are found within the tissue. Integrins are proteins that are thought to aid in implantation, so if the integrins are absent, it may explain why you are not getting pregnant. Integrin expression and its relevance in conception is still somewhat controversial. More studies are necessary to flesh out the exact role of integrins in the uterine lining.

Sonohystogram/Uterine Sounding

You can think of your sonohystogram and sounding procedure as a mock embryo transfer. The purpose is to take a thorough look at your uterus and make sure that there aren't any fibroids or anything else blocking the cavity and impeding the transfer. Because of the extreme time-sensitivity of IVF, your doctor wants to make absolutely sure that when it comes time for your embryos to be transferred, your uterus is able to receive them.

The doctor will insert a small catheter through the cervix and into the uterus. With an ultrasound, he will use small gradations on the catheter to determine the depth that is best for transfer. There is a precise location where the embryos should be deposited; knowing the depth at which to place the catheter will make your transfer go much smoother. He will then instill a little bit of sterile water into the uterus to help him see the cavity and make sure there is nothing occluding it. He'll also take a measurement of your uterus, which tells him exactly where to put the embryos on transfer day.

FACT

The cervix is so narrow, or stenotic, in some women that the catheter cannot get through. While this is easily fixed through a very minor surgical procedure, you don't want to find this out on the day of your transfer.

You may notice a small amount of cramping during the procedure. If your cervix is particularly narrow, that cramping may be more intense. If you are concerned about the pain, take 1000mg of Tylenol (two extra strength tablets) about two hours before your test. The cramping should dissipate once the test is finished, usually in a matter of minutes.

Surgical Procedures

Surgeries to help with diagnosing or addressing fertility problems have come a long way in recent years. While surgery is not for everyone or every fertility problem, it can be an important part of your fertility process. Surgery can be used in two main ways—to help diagnose fertility problems or issues, or as a tool to treat an existing fertility problem.

Hysteroscopy

Hysteroscopy is a relatively minor surgical procedure that can be used both to diagnose and treat problems associated with your uterus. A basic hysteroscopy involves inserting into your uterus a small tube with an optical device attached to the end. Once this tube is inserted, your uterus is distended with fluid to help doctors get a better view. This can help find problems like a uterine septum, polyps, fibroids, scarring, or adhesions of your uterus. Sometimes hysteroscopy can also be used to see problems with obstruction at the uterine end of the Fallopian tubes.

This is generally an outpatient procedure. It can be done in a hospital, surgical center, or potentially even in the office setting. Your doctor will help you decide where the best location is if you decide that a hysteroscopy is a good plan of treatment for your particular case.

The anesthesia used for your hysteroscopy will largely be determined by the purpose of the hysteroscopy. General anesthesia is typically used if the hysteroscopy is being done to treat a problem. Local anesthesia is used if it is done in the office setting or if it is being done purely for diagnostic purposes.

Your hysteroscopy can take as little as five minutes if the purpose is simply to look around the uterine cavity. If treatment or additional procedures are done, it can take longer. Even with treatments, a hysteroscopy is generally about a thirty-minute procedure.

Your physician may decide that a hysteroscopic procedure is beneficial if you suffer from repeated miscarriages or are having trouble conceiving and she suspects a uterine problem. Uterine problems might include adhesions, a uterine septum, fibroids, endometrial polyps, and so forth. If it is found that you have adhesions or other uterine blockages, a hysteroscopy can be a great, noninvasive way to try to treat these problems.

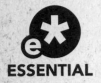

ESSENTIAL

One of the best things that hysteroscopy has going for it is that is a very minimally invasive procedure performed without incisions. For you, the good news is that the lack of incisions means fewer risks of future problems caused by the actual procedure, like scarring and adhesions, which can affect your fertility.

If you have any questions about the use of hysteroscopy in your treatment, be sure to talk to your fertility specialist or other practitioner about its use. Most women don't have many problems with the procedure, but cramping can last for a few hours afterwards and you may experience some bleeding. If you used a general anesthesia you will need to take the rest of the day off to recover from the drug; otherwise, you may be able to head right back to your normal life. A few other risks are involved but are much less likely, such as infection and perforation of the uterine cavity.

Laparoscopy

This surgical type of testing will require the use of a surgical center or hospital. It is a more advanced type of fertility testing. When other testing has proven unhelpful or inconclusive, surgery via a laparoscope may be your next option.

Your doctor uses this surgery to help visualize problems in your abdomen, uterus, or ovaries. She may be able to find problems that other less invasive tests could not find. Or the surgery may be used to confirm your diagnosis of several issues. It may also be used to diagnose and immediately treat issues.

Prior to surgery, you and your care provider will probably discuss what will happen during the surgery. This may include how to treat problems that are identified during this surgery. The benefit of this is that you will not require a second surgery to do the treatments. Be sure to discuss the limitations of this surgery with your doctor.

MRI

Magnetic resonance imaging (MRI) can be a helpful diagnostic aid. Sometimes a persistently elevated prolactin level can indicate a benign growth on the pituitary gland that is causing it to pump out extra hormones; an MRI can help look for that tumor. This sounds really scary, but it is not cancer and chances are the tumor just needs to be treated with medication. In fact, it has been estimated that about 25 percent of the American population have small pituitary tumors; of those tumors, almost 40 percent secrete prolactin. A majority of those tumors don't even need to be treated, but depending on the whole clinical picture, medication is often the first choice if yours requires therapy.

If one of the sonograms shows that there might be an abnormal wall in the uterus or other abnormal structure in the pelvis, having an MRI can help your doctor better visualize what it might be. This is definitely not appropriate for everyone undergoing infertility treatment, but it is a useful adjunct to the diagnostic process.

Preimplantation Genetic Diagnosis (PGD)

If genetic problems are part of your inability to conceive naturally, you may be interested in taking genetic testing one step further than typical procedure done via amniocentesis. Preimplantation genetic diagnosis (PGD) can be done with assisted reproductive technologies (ART), like IVF. This procedure involves running genetic tests on the embryos before they are placed inside your body for possible implantation.

PGD is an involved procedure and can be quite expensive, particularly because it is not usually covered by insurance. Embryos are created using IVF and are allowed to grow in the lab for a few days. On the third day following the retrieval, a PGD specialist will remove one cell from each embryo. The cells are shipped to a specialized lab that will biopsy each cell and look at the chromosomes. Any abnormalities are reported to your clinic, where you will be given the results. Genetically normal embryos can be transferred; genetically abnormal embryos are then discarded.

This can be helpful when you know that you and your partner both carry the gene for a genetic disorder, like cystic fibrosis, to ensure that your child does not actually have the disease. It can also be a helpful diagnostic tool when you are not sure what is causing your infertility and the doctor suspects that it may be genetic in nature.

FACT

PGD can also be used in fertile couples for gender selection. The use of this practice is quite controversial, so as a result, not many clinics offer this service. If they do, often they'll perform it in limited circumstances. If you are interested in this, check to make sure that your clinic performs this testing when you make the appointment.

Though small, there is always a risk when you tamper with an embryo. To minimize this risk, make sure to find an embryologist who has a great deal of experience performing this procedure before moving forward.

CHAPTER 10

What to Expect from Infertility Treatment

Infertility treatment is like nothing you've ever experienced before. You'll see the doctor and clinic staff more than you'll see your best friends. You'll speak with the nurses on a daily basis and have frequent blood draws and ultrasound appointments. And then suddenly, you'll get a call one day that you may need to reschedule your plans for the next few days because you're ready for insemination or egg retrieval. Having an idea of what to expect can make the process much easier.

Process Overview

Undergoing infertility treatment is a unique process, to say the least. Once the doctor chooses a medication regimen for you, you will most likely sit down with a nurse, either in a group setting or individually, who will explain the protocol, the medications, and most importantly, how to administer them. She will also discuss the policies of the facility, including the hours that you can come in for monitoring, what phone numbers to call if you have a questions, and how you are supposed to handle medication emergencies after hours. If the nurse does not address these issues, they are important questions that you should ask during this appointment.

There are many different regimens and approaches to treatment. Your reproductive endocrinologist (RE) will start with the simplest treatment plan that gives you the best chance for pregnancy. This could mean an oral medication like Clomid, or even IVF.

Taking Medication

Whatever protocol is selected for you, you will follow the instructions given to you by the nursing staff. The nurses act as a liaison between you and your doctor during treatment, relaying instructions from the doctor to you. It is common for you to be in for monitoring on a regular basis, often every day if you are being treated with IVF. Don't worry; this frequent monitoring doesn't usually last more than two weeks.

Depending on what type of ovarian stimulation you're taking, you may need a final injection of a form of human chorionic gonadotropin (hCG), which will help your eggs complete their maturation. Once you take this injection, ovulation will occur approximately thirty-six hours later. Either your insemination or egg retrieval will be scheduled according to the time they tell you to take the injection. Sometimes, if your partner's semen analysis is normal, the doctor may just instruct you when you have sex. You may need additional hormonal support during the luteal phase of your cycle, i.e., after you ovulate.

When Will I Find Out If It Worked?

Finally, after about two weeks, you will need to take a pregnancy test. You may be able to test at home using a urine pregnancy test, or you may be asked to come back into the office for a blood test. It is really important to not take your pregnancy test earlier then recommended. Some of the medications, namely the trigger injection, will cause the test to read falsely positive.

If you are pregnant, most REs will follow your pregnancy through the first several weeks. Once a heartbeat can be seen on the ultrasound and your RE feels comfortable with the success of your pregnancy, usually around ten weeks, you will be discharged and sent to your regular ob/gyn for routine prenatal care.

What If It Doesn't Work?

If you are not pregnant, your doctor will analyze your entire cycle from your response to the medication to the results of your hormonal blood tests. A plan will be created for your next cycle. If it does not work the first, second, or even third time, it doesn't mean that you won't get pregnant. Don't lose hope!

Monitoring

Monitoring is an integral part of fertility treatment. Whether you are having IUIs, going through IVF, or even using donated eggs or sperm, the doctor will need to assess your ovaries, uterus, and hormone levels fairly frequently, sometimes every day.

ALERT

Make sure that you have a voicemail system or answering machine set up so that you can receive your instructions when you are not available to answer the phone. Most likely, your instructions will be for later that night, so it is really important that you receive them in a timely fashion.

The doctor will make a decision on the basis of those results, and you'll get your instructions later in the day. This is why it's very important that the travel time to your clinic is reasonable; you'll be making the trip a lot.

Estradiol

Estradiol is a form of estrogen and is secreted by the developing egg follicle(s). As the follicle grows and the egg matures, your estradiol level increases as well. In the very beginning of your menstrual cycle, your estradiol levels are low, usually under 60ng/ml. By the time the egg has reached maturity, your estradiol level will be above 200ng/ml. This is true for every egg follicle on the ovary. So if you are being treated with IVF with the goal of producing many egg follicles, your estradiol level could easily be several thousand ng/ml. If you are taking medication before having insemination, your estradiol level will not be quite so high, but will still be several hundred ng/ml.

Your doctor will want to monitor your estradiol very closely. Each clinic will have its own criteria for how they want the estradiol level to rise, and will adjust your medication based on the result of your testing accordingly. Your risk for serious complications increases if your estradiol gets too high, so it is extremely important that you follow your clinic's instructions very closely.

LH

As you now know, a rise in your luteinizing hormone (LH) levels precedes ovulation. So if your doctor sees that your LH level is suddenly starting to rise, it may indicate that your body is getting ready to ovulate. Once an egg follicle starts to reach maturity, it will trigger the LH surge. This isn't such a big deal if you are undergoing insemination or will be having intercourse because you don't want a high number of eggs released. But if you are going through IVF, the goal is to produce many eggs. These eggs will be at different levels of maturity, so you don't want the lead follicle to trigger ovulation when the remainder of the eggs isn't quite mature yet. This is why you'll be taking a suppressive medication to prevent you from ovulating.

Progesterone

Just as the LH surge can predict ovulation, your progesterone level will also start to increase just prior to ovulation. So if your blood results show that your ovulation is approaching 3ng/ml (usually the point where ovulation is presumed to occur), they can prepare you for retrieval or insemination if you are ready.

Your physician may also check your progesterone periodically during the diagnostic phase to determine if you are ovulating on your own.

ESSENTIAL

If your progesterone level indicates that you've ovulated and you're going through IVF, your cycle will likely need to be cancelled. Once eggs are released from the ovary, it is not possible to retrieve them from the abdomen or Fallopian tube. No further treatment is possible at that point.

Ultrasound

Ultrasound is often thought of as being beneficial for pregnancy, but you may not know that ultrasound plays a large part in most fertility treatment programs. You will get to know the ultrasound technicians at your fertility clinic very well.

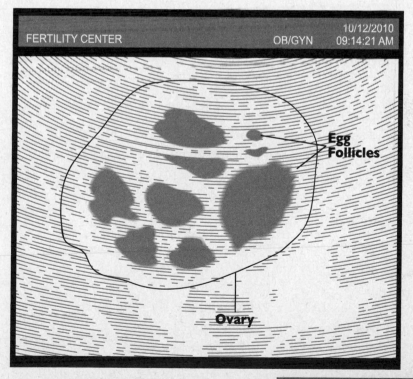

A follicular ultrasound

By using mostly transvaginal ultrasound, meaning that a probe is inserted into the vagina for better views of your reproductive organs, doctors can see the cervix, your uterus, ovaries, endometrial (uterine) lining, and even down to the fine detail of follicle production.

During different phases of your cycle, ultrasound can be used to monitor what is going on inside your body. Your fertility team can monitor how your follicles grow in relation to your hormonal production or in reaction to medications given. This can help your doctor adjust medications as needed to help you to maximize your response. Using ultrasound in this manner can also help prevent overmedication and risking your health.

The endometrial or uterine lining can also be looked at in great detail. Your uterine lining will be monitored for thickness at various points in your cycle. Since it responds to various hormones to build a secure place for implantation of your fertilized egg, it is a vital component on the road to pregnancy. You may need to take hormone supplements to help you build a thicker lining that will support a pregnancy.

Lastly, ultrasound can be used to help diagnose any abnormalities of the uterus, ovaries, or Fallopian tubes. This may be something like endometriosis, cysts, fibroids, and any structural abnormality. It can also help suggest that further testing is needed based on suspicious information revealed.

Hormone Supplementation

Supplemental medications can be nearly anything that addresses an issue you need help with during your fertility treatment. Some medications might be used to help you correct certain hormonal imbalances, while others are prescribed to manage blood-clotting issues found during testing.

FACT

Remember that these medications can affect urine and blood pregnancy tests. When undergoing assisted reproductive technology like superovulation and IVF, don't be tempted to take a pregnancy test without your doctor's okay. You may get inaccurate results.

During the course of your treatment, you and your reproductive specialty team will decide on a medication protocol. This protocol will go along with your known fertility issues. Except in a few rare instances, you will start at the lowest dose, strength, and type of medication possible in order to minimize the risk of complications with any given medication.

Your team may decide from the beginning of treatment that supplemental medication is required for a successful cycle, or it may not be until mid-cycle that your team makes a change or addition to your medications to help ensure a successful and safe cycle. Which medications, if any, are used for supplementation depend on many factors.

Estrogen Supplementation

During the course of your fertility treatment, your blood work will be monitored as well as your uterine lining. If it is determined that you need to boost your estrogen levels, you may be asked to take supplemental estrogen. This is usually, and thankfully, done in patch form. This means you simply wear a small piece of plastic tape that has the estrogen imbedded in it. The medication is absorbed through your skin. No muss, no fuss!

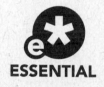

ESSENTIAL

Some people have an allergy to the tape or adhesive on the patch. Make sure to let your clinic know if you have any irritation, itchiness, redness, or swelling. They will need to switch you to a different form of estrogen.

In addition to the patch, you can also take estrogen supplementation in pill form. These are taken either orally or inserted into the vagina. It is the same pill, but just taken via a different route.

Progesterone Supplementation

Progesterone supplementation can be used in high-level fertility procedures like IVF and superovulation. It can also be used to help supplement some other women and is commonly used in cases of frequent or recurrent pregnancy loss and for unexplained infertility. This is most often done as an injectable form or as a vaginal suppository. The injectables are usually suspended in oil and are given intramuscularly.

Mixing Your Medication

You will want to follow the specific directions for each medication when you actually draw up or mix your drugs. This will be given to you before you start your medication therapy. It may be gone over in a class setting as well.

Drawing Back a Premixed Medication

Start with a clean surface and clean hands. Wipe off the tops of any vials of medication with alcohol swabs. Inject the vial with your needle, and invert the vial so that it is upside down. With the needle completely covered in the fluid, draw the exact amount of medication you need. Remove the needle from the vial and, with needle pointed in the air, flick the syringe to move air bubbles to the top. Squeeze slightly on the plunge to remove excess air. Now you'll recap your needle in preparation to inject the medications.

Mixing Powdered Medication

If your medication doesn't come premixed, you will actually need to mix the diluents, or liquid, into the powder. It is very important to only use the recommended or included liquid when mixing your medication—if you don't, the medication may not work properly.

First, prepare all of your supplies:

- Alcohol wipes
- Needle and syringe
- Bottle of medication (the powder)
- Diluent (liquid)

Next, remove all of the caps from the bottles and swab with an alcohol pad. Put the needle into the rubber stopper of the bottle of diluent. Turn the bottle upside down so the tip of the needle is facing upward and is in the liquid solution. Draw back the amount of solution necessary to mix your medication, usually 1ml to 2ml. Remove the needle from the bottle of diluent, and push the needle into the bottle of powder. Depress the plunger to inject the liquid into the powder and watch it dissolve. You can shake the bottle a little bit to make sure everything dissolves. Turn the bottle back upside down, and pull back the plunger to remove the mixed medication.

FACT

Some medications, like Bravelle and Menopur, require that you mix several vials of powder into 1ml of solution. When doing so you may not be able to retrieve every drop from the vial. This is fine; do not panic.

You can change the actual needle and put a fresh one on once you've mixed the medication. A sharper needle will make the injection a little easier and less painful.

Subcutaneous Injections

A subcutaneous injection is given just under the surface of the skin. These can be given in the thigh or abdomen and are therefore easier to give yourself than intramuscular injections.

Again, you should always begin by washing your hands. Choose a location to give your injection where you have plenty of room and quiet time. Then gather your supplies. You will need:

- Alcohol wipes
- Medications
- Syringes
- Sharps container

Once you have your medications ready and drawn up, you will select a site.

The best bets for subcutaneous injection sites are the abdomen (belly) and thigh. These work well for most people. You can also give yourself these injections easily.

Example of a subcutaneous injection site

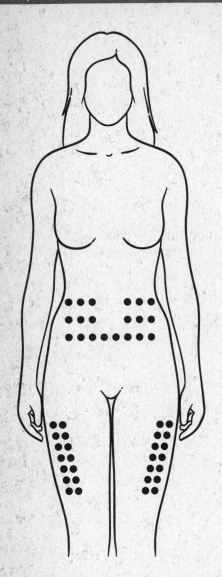

Select a site and wipe it with the alcohol swab—remember not to get closer than two inches around the belly button or navel. Pinch the area of skin you intend to use. Holding the syringe like a pencil, press the needle quickly into your skin at a 90 degree angle. Hold the syringe firmly to prevent the needle from bouncing off your skin. Depress the plunger and administer all of the medication. Remember to always discard your used needles into your sharps container—a special plastic container that prevents the needles from poking out of the container, thereby preventing accidental punctures from used needles—and never into the garbage. Hold or massage the site for pain relief.

Remember that different medications, while administered with the same technique, will feel differently when you inject them. The same may be said of other medications given by someone else, like your partner. Practicing will help with any fear and anxiety you or your partner may have.

Remember to put the needle in—long or short—quickly. This will make the injection portion nearly painless if you do it rapidly enough. Also, depress the plunger slowly. This can be difficult if you are nervous, but the more slowly you inject the liquids, the less pain you will feel. By doing it slowly you allow time for the tissues to stretch.

ESSENTIAL

You should always mix your medications before cleansing your medication site. Have the syringe ready to give the injection so that you have that part out of way.

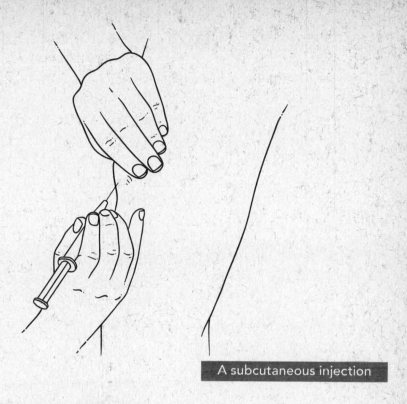

A subcutaneous injection

Intramuscular Injections

An intramuscular (IM) injection means that you will be giving an injection into a muscle. This is used for a variety of medications, including progesterone and human chorionic gonadotrophin.

You should always begin by washing your hands. Choose a location to give your injection where you have plenty of room and quiet time. Be sure that the location is clean as well. Then gather your supplies. You will need:

- Alcohol wipes
- Medications
- Syringes
- Sharps container

You will choose a spot for the injection to be given. Divide each buttock into four quadrants. You will want to inject into the upper, outer quadrant of your buttocks, almost toward the hipbone. If you choose the buttocks, you will probably want someone else to help you. Pinch a hunk of the muscle between your thumb and forefinger to test your location, making certain the spot isn't already sore from a previous injection.

Once you have decided on a spot, open your alcohol wipe and cleanse the area to be injected, as well as the top of the vial. Allow this area to dry, or the injection will be more painful.

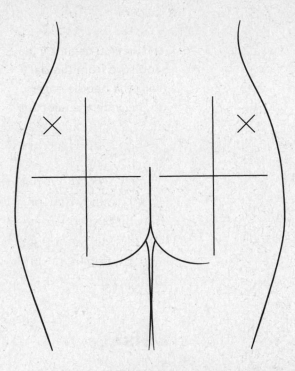

Example of an intramuscular injection site

When the area is dry, take your weight off the side you've chosen as your injection site by either lying down or taking the weight off that foot—this makes it easier to give the injection. Stretch the area of skin between your fingers, and hold it tightly enough that it doesn't move.

Take your needle and insert it all the way until none of the needle is showing. Pull back slightly on the plunger of the syringe. You should not see blood. If you do see blood, you have hit a blood vessel and must remove the needle entirely and start over.

If there is no blood returned in the syringe, depress the plunger and inject the medications. When you are done, pull the needle straight out. If you experience a bit of bleeding, and there should not be much of it, use the alcohol pad to put a bit of pressure on the spot until the bleeding has stopped. You can also massage the injection site gently for pain relief and apply a heating pad for a few minutes. The heat and massage will help the medication be absorbed into the muscle.

FACT

You should rotate which side you use for injections. This will help prevent you from getting too sore from the daily injections. You should also rotate the spot where the needle enters. This is easier to do if someone else is helping you with the injections.

When you are done with the needle it needs to go into a sharps container. Your fertility clinic or pharmacy may provide one for you, or you can purchase one yourself. You might also use something handy from home, like a detergent bottle with a screw cap lid or other heavy plastic bottle or container. Return any sharps containers or other used needles to your doctor or pharmacy for proper disposal.

Complications and Risks

Infertility treatment isn't inherently dangerous or life threatening, but it can cause serious complications if your cycle isn't monitored properly. It is really important to keep track of how you are feeling and ask your nurse if you are concerned about anything. Some of the medications can cause alarming side effects, like visual problems, that need to be addressed. Don't ever hesitate to mention anything you are concerned about—even seemingly minor complaints may be important.

Ovarian Torsion

This is one of the rarest complications resulting from infertility treatment. As you progress through a medicated cycle, your ovaries tend to enlarge slightly. Of course, with IVF your ovaries will get significantly larger than if you are going through an insemination cycle. If the ovaries get large and heavy enough, it could cause one of the ligaments holding it in place to twist over on itself. If that were to happen, blood flow to the ovary would be cut off, causing the ovary to die if the ovarian ligament were not untwisted quickly.

If you develop ovarian torsion, you would feel sudden and extreme abdominal pain. It would likely worsen over time and you may become nauseated or even vomit. Anytime you have a lot of abdominal or pelvic pain, you should call your doctor, or the on-call service if there is one available.

If the doctor suspects that you have ovarian torsion and recommends that you go to the hospital, it is better that you go to the one where your doctor is licensed to practice. Your doctor will be able to expedite your care through the emergency room and into surgery much quicker than if you are in a hospital where he doesn't have privileges. That being said, if that hospital is several hours away, you should proceed to the nearest emergency room instead.

The best way to prevent this is to rest as much as you can while you are cycling, especially once you are finished with your medication and waiting to take your pregnancy test. This is when your ovaries are at their largest and you are at the greatest risk.

Ovarian Hyperstimulation Syndrome

Stimulation of the ovaries can cause ovarian hyperstimulation syndrome (OHSS), a situation in which your ovaries enlarge drastically and leak fluid into the abdomen. This can cause pain, bloating, weight gain, shortness of breath, dizziness, nausea, and vomiting. The first sign is significant weight gain and bloating in a short amount of time. Make sure to call your doctor if you have any symptoms.

You are at the greatest risk for OHSS right after ovulation (or egg retrieval) up until your pregnancy test. Young, thin women with a high response to the stimulant medication have a slightly higher tendency to become hyperstimulated, but it can affect women of all ages and sizes.

Pregnancy can actually make this problem worse because your hormone levels stay high, instead of declining as they normally would once you would get your period.

Treatment varies according to the severity of the syndrome. Most mild to moderate cases are treated simply with bed rest for a short period of time until your ovaries return to their normal size. If it progresses to the severe form, you may require hospitalization or intravenous medication.

FACT

Weighing yourself every day once you start cycling can be an easy way to monitor for OHSS, as you will likely see this weight gain much sooner than if you hadn't kept track of your weight. Weigh yourself, undressed, at the same time each morning. Make sure to report significant weight gain in a twenty-four hour period.

Multi-Fetal Pregnancy

The rate of multiple pregnancies is on the rise. Some of this is due to the rates of assisted reproductive technology and other fertility treatments. Of course, it is still possible to get pregnant with multiples using any fertility treatment. The rate of twinning is about one in every eighty-nine pregnancies.

What if you find out that you are having more than one baby? Twins are the most common form of multiple pregnancy. While there are increased risks if you are having twins, many practitioners still consider you a candidate for a normal birth while being more closely monitored. If you are having higher order multiples—triplets or more—you will probably wish to seek out the care of a perinatologist who specializes in multiple pregnancy.

You will want to ask questions about how your practitioner handles multiple pregnancies.

- What type of extra monitoring, if any, will I have?
- What considerations will be made at the birth?
- What is your Cesarean rate for multiples?
- When would you consider doing a Cesarean delivery?
- What type of routine interventions do you use in multiple births?
- Will I be able to breastfeed my babies right away?

It is worth having a discussion with you partner about how you feel about having multiples. If that is something you don't feel comfortable with, you need to convey this to your RE. He can proceed much more conservatively with your treatment or even recommend only transferring a single embryo during IVF, instead of the usual two or three.

Do Fertility Drugs Cause Cancer?

Some initial studies did point to a possible connection between infertility drugs and cancer. It is important to know, however, that certain causes of infertility can increase your risk for cancer as well. For example, PCOS can increase your risk for endometrial cancer. In fact, never giving birth can also increase your risk for certain types of cancer. These early studies did not take that fact into account. So it is unclear whether the observed cancer risk is a result of the infertility drugs, or the cause of the infertility itself. Current studies do not show any link between taking fertility drugs and your risk for developing breast, uterine, or ovarian cancer. However, more studies are definitely needed to confirm this.

After all of this, there are still more questions to ask! You can never ask too many questions. Don't worry about being annoying or causing trouble; these practices and the people who staff them understand that you are investing your emotional and fertile future with them. They are willing to answer questions to help you make a choice.

CHAPTER 11

Medications

There's a good chance you'll be taking some form of medication while undergoing your treatment. The doctor will likely start you on the simplest regimen appropriate to your diagnosis and give it a few cycles. If you still aren't pregnant, she'll make a decision about moving to the next step and try that for a few cycles. Don't be surprised if it takes a couple of cycles to determine which one is best. Remember that everyone responds differently to the medication and it may just take some time to find the best one for you.

Oral Ovulation Induction

These pills are the easiest protocol used to induce ovulation. If you know that you are anovulatory, they are the usual first try. Clomid and Letrazole work by inhibiting your estrogen levels. Your pituitary gland pumps out more FSH and LH when your estrogen level is low, similar to the beginning of your menstrual cycle. The additional follicle stimulating hormone (FSH) and luteinizing hormone (LH) encourages follicular growth in the ovaries.

Clomid

Clomid is a pill that you take by mouth every day for five days. Doses range from 50mg to 150mg or even 200mg (one to four pills, at the same time each day). You will be instructed to take your first dose in the beginning of your cycle, usually on day three or day five. Once you have finished taking your pills, the doctor may recommend having periodic ultrasounds or blood work done. The other option is that the doctor may recommend you use an ovulation predictor kit to check for ovulation, and then begin having intercourse with the positive result.

Letrazole

Letrazole works in a similar fashion to Clomid. However, Clomid can inhibit the development of your uterine lining and your cervical mucus. If your doctor notices a thin endometrium during an ultrasound, she can either supplement you with additional estrogen to help counteract the effect of the Clomid, or recommend the use of Letrazole during your next cycle. Letrazole doesn't typically produce this same inhibitory response on your uterine lining that Clomid does.

Letrazole is taken in a similar manner to Clomid—one or two pills at the same time, every day for five days in the beginning of your cycle. You may be periodically monitored or asked to check at home for your ovulation. Once your follicles are ready, you'll be instructed to either have intercourse or return to the office for insemination.

Injectable Gonadotropins

If the oral medications don't work, or your doctor recommends moving directly to injectable gonadotropins or IVF, you will be taking a synthetic form of hormones your body naturally produces, namely FSH and LH. Boosting the level of these hormones causes your body to increase the number of egg follicles that are developing in the ovary.

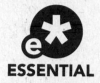

ESSENTIAL

It can be helpful to determine the extent of your medication coverage before you begin infertility treatment. Talking to your doctor, nurse, or billing associate about your coverage up front can help you maximize your coverage and minimize the amount of money you need to pay.

Which medication you use will depend on the number of eggs desired, your body's hormonal response to the medications, the procedure you are undergoing, and your physician's preference for medications—just to name a few.

It's not unusual to be taking FSH alone, both FSH and human menopausal gonadotropin (hMG) together, or hMG alone. Your doctor will select the best medication protocol for you.

FSH

There are several brands of FSH on the market right now, including:

- Bravelle
- Follistim
- Gonal-F

These brands are all similar, but your physician may have a preference based on his personal experiences. You may also have insurance coverage on one form, which should be factored in to the medication you are prescribed.

They are all taken as a subcutaneous injection, though each is prepared and mixed in a different manner. Follistim and Gonal F both come as a preloaded pen or as individual vials of medication that require mixing.

ALERT

Once you start taking your stimulation, double check that you have your final trigger injection. Keep it in a safe place where you won't forget it. You don't want to realize that you've misplaced it once you've been instructed to take it. It can be difficult to find a late night pharmacy that carries what you need.

HMG

Human menopausal gonadotropin, or hMG, is a combination of both FSH and LH. The two most common brands are Menopur and Repronex, though Pergonal is sometimes used as well. Again, your doctor will recommend which one he thinks is the best fit for you.

The Trigger Shot

Your trigger shot is the final injection that you'll take prior to your insemination or egg retrieval. It is usually a form of human chorionic gonadotropin, or hCG. The hCG causes the eggs within the follicles to complete their maturation and prepare for ovulation. Unlike the rest of the stimulation, you will likely be given a specific time to take the injection.

Ovidrel

Ovidrel is a lower dose of hCG and is usually given during ovulation induction cycles for insemination or intercourse. You may not even need to take it if you ovulate on your own, depending on what your doctor recommends. Because you'll know exactly when you're ovulating, taking Ovidrel can also help with timing insemination more precisely.

Ovidrel comes in a prefilled syringe. Simply open the packaging and dispel any extra air in the syringe. Do this by removing the cap on the needle and holding it so the needle is pointing upwards. Gently tap on the syringe to move the air bubbles to the top of the syringe. Then, lightly press on the plunger until the air has been removed from the syringe.

ALERT

Ovidrel and hCG are both detected by urine pregnancy tests. Make sure to wait at least a full two weeks from when you inject it before you take a pregnancy test. Any earlier, and you will likely have a false positive result.

Once the medicine has been prepared, you can inject the medication subcutaneously into the front part of your thigh or lower abdomen.

hCG (Novarel/Pregnyl)

If you are going through IVF, you will need to take hCG as your final trigger injection. As it will cause ovulation around thirty-six hours later, it is very closely timed according to when your egg retrieval will be. Make sure that you take it on time. If you take it too early, your eggs might not be fully mature once they are retrieved. If you take it too late, there is a strong possibility that you may ovulate prior to your egg retrieval. If this happens, your cycle will likely be canceled, as there is nothing your physician can do to remove your eggs once they've been removed from the ovary.

Ovarian Suppression

If you are undergoing IVF, or the doctor finds that you have a tendency to ovulate prematurely, your RE might recommend that you suppress your ovaries' natural inclination to ovulate. This gives your doctor control over how much FSH and LH your ovaries are exposed to. He can be very precise when it comes to your stimulation, allowing you to have a better ovarian response.

Lupron

Lupron is a gonadotropin releasing hormone (GnRH) agonist, meaning that at first it signals your pituitary gland to release a lot of FSH and LH. After about five days, your pituitary becomes incapable of releasing any FSH or LH. This helps prevent an LH surge during your cycle, which in turn prevents you from ovulating prematurely. Your medical team can control your hormonal output with other medications to time everything very closely to allow the maximum number of high-quality eggs to be retrieved exactly when they are ready. Lupron is usually started in the luteal phase of the preceding cycle.

It is injected subcutaneously, into the fatty tissue under the skin of the front part of your thighs or the lower part of your abdomen. You'll begin taking this a few days after you ovulate, through your period and into the follicular phase of your next cycle. Your doctor will instruct you when to stop taking it, usually right before your egg retrieval.

ALERT

You will only take Antagon OR Lupron, not both of them. The doctor makes the decision based on your age, diagnosis, and anticipated stimulation. Sometimes, the selected medication may not be the best choice because of your response. Your RE can't predict your response ahead of time and may need to put you on an alternate protocol with your next cycle.

The most common side effects of taking Lupron are headaches, hot flashes, and irritability. These tend to be more pronounced if you are taking Lupron for several weeks without any other medication, like your stimulation or estrogen supplements. Lupron puts your body into a state similar to menopause, keeping your estrogen levels low. The symptoms usually are alleviated once you add on the other medications, because they will raise your estrogen level.

Ganirelix

Ganirelix, or Antagon, is a GnRH antagonist. This means that it shuts down your body's natural production of FSH and LH. This also prevents the

LH surge, which triggers ovulation. This medication is a little different than Lupron because you will typically begin taking Antagon once you've started your stimulation, usually once a dominant follicle has been identified. Your doctor will instruct you when to begin taking it.

This medication comes as a prefilled syringe, meaning that the medication has already been mixed and loaded into the syringe with a needle attached. All you need to do is open the packaging and inject the medication subcutaneously. You will inject one syringe every night or as instructed by your RE.

Other Medications

Supplemental medications can be nearly anything that addresses an issue that you need help with during your fertility treatment. These medications can encourage implantation, prevent infection, and reduce swelling and inflammation.

Baby Aspirin

Baby aspirin is given to women who have blood-clotting disorders or may have had problems with placental perfusion in previous pregnancies. It is also given to combat some autoimmune disorders, which cause your body to attack a pregnancy as a foreign substance. This oral medication can be taken temporarily in the early weeks of pregnancy or continuously throughout pregnancy. However, it may be advised that you discontinue its use in the third trimester of pregnancy for fear of bleeding problems during the birth.

The Birth Control Pill

The doctor may instruct you to take the birth control pill for one month before your cycle starts. It may sound completely counterintuitive to be taking the birth control pill when you are trying to get pregnant, but the pill does have a few benefits when taking it during infertility treatment.

First, it gives the doctor control over when you will get your period. You'll take the twenty-one days of active pills and usually get a period a few days after you finish taking them. Sometimes the doctor may have you extend the number of active pills you take in order to delay your period. This is particularly helpful if you need to give your employer notice of when you'll be out of work, or if you have a religious obligation that you need to work around.

The pill also keeps your hormone levels low for the month leading to your cycle. This offers extra suppressive action during the month that you are actually stimulating. It is not appropriate for everyone, especially older women who may not stimulate as well.

Medrol

Medrol, or methylprednisolone, is a mild steroid that you may need to take after having an egg retrieval. It helps reduce any post-operative inflammation and assists in implantation. It's generally taken one to two times a day beginning the night of the egg retrieval. You will take it for approximately four days, or as directed by your doctor.

An Antibiotic

If you are undergoing IVF, you will need a short course of antibiotics to prevent infection after the egg retrieval. Despite all of the standard precautions, infection is still a risk after any surgical procedure.

ALERT

Ask your doctor or pharmacist about how to take the antibiotic. Some commonly prescribed drugs can cause nausea or other stomach upset. Make sure to clarify the instructions so the medication works properly.

Given that the doctor will be transferring embryos back into the uterine cavity within a few days, it is of the utmost importance that any potential for infection be eliminated.

Viagra

Here's a new one to many people: women's use of the medication Viagra. The way that Viagra works on everyone is that it helps blood flow to capillaries, causing certain parts of the body to have increased blood flow. Some fertility centers are using this medication to help increase blood flow to the uterus. It is used as a suppository to be inserted vaginally.

Medications for Men

You will undoubtedly be taking the majority of the medication when undergoing infertility treatment. But there are medications that your partner should be taking as well. It's standard treatment that your partner should take a course of antibiotics prior to producing his sperm for IVF. The lab will need to make sure that they are receiving a clean specimen and that bacteria found in the sperm won't contaminate the rest of the embryos and sperm samples.

Vitamins

Vitamins are a common treatment in sperm-related issues. For a long time it was standard issue to give vitamin B_{12} injections to men in fertility treatments. It has been found to increase the number of quality sperm in some men. Studies have found that folic acid can also affect the sperm counts of many men. This means that your partner needs to be taking his vitamins as well to ensure proper sperm counts with healthy sperm.

Antibiotics

Sometimes a problem with sperm production may be caused by an infection in your partner's body that may not even have any outward symptoms. This type of problem is usually treated with antibiotics, which may be given as an oral regimen or by injection. A normal course of antibiotics is about ten days long, though some infections may require longer or stronger treatment. Your or your partner's doctor can help you find what treatment is right for you.

Medication Emergencies

Medication emergencies can and do happen at any point. Perhaps you have broken an ampoule of your medications. Maybe your doctor has increased or changed your medications, and it is late at night and you are stuck without enough.

Never hesitate to call the doctor on call to ask what to do. Your fertility clinic may have an emergency kit of medications on hand that they can get to you immediately.

When choosing your fertility clinic, be sure to ask what their policy is on medication emergencies. There may be a specific coordinator to call, or you may just call the line for regular emergencies. Do not despair if you find yourself in this situation.

CHAPTER 12

Insemination

Insemination is an older form of treatment that can be very successful in helping you overcome certain fertility barriers. Because it is less invasive, less costly, and can be done with greater ease, most couples with fertility problems try it at one point or another over the course of their treatment.

What Is Artificial Insemination?

Artificial insemination is a process where sperm is collected, washed, and then inserted through a small catheter directly into the female reproductive tract. It's usually fairly inexpensive, and is often covered by insurance. In fact, some policies will even require that a certain number of insemination cycles be attempted before you can be covered for more aggressive treatment like IVF.

Insemination should be done right around the time of ovulation so that the sperm cells have a greater chance of encountering the egg once it's released. This procedure can be done with or without the use of medications to boost your ovulatory response. Each clinic will have their own policy, but having one or two inseminations before and/or after ovulation is pretty standard. The sperm can be inseminated directly into the uterus, or right around the cervical os (opening).

The success rates for insemination vary widely depending on a lot of factors: your partner's sperm count, your response to the medications, your age, and your diagnosis, just to name a few. Studies looking at the success rates of IUI report conflicting results. Some studies put the average success rate at around 8 percent, while others estimate the success rate at 20 percent. Generally speaking though, your success rate will be higher with a younger maternal age and higher sperm count. Taking ovulation induction medication also slightly raises your chance of success.

Intrauterine Insemination (IUI)

Intrauterine insemination (IUI) is the more common of the two insemination procedures and is now the gold standard of artificial inseminations. This process is used for many different causes of infertility and has a varying pregnancy rate, from about 5–25 percent per cycle, depending on the diagnosis and protocol used. It may or may not include the use of medications. In this procedure, the washed sperm will be injected directly into the uterus through a small catheter inserted through the cervix.

Intracervical Insemination (ICI)

Intracervical inseminations are not done as frequently now as they once were. Now that the technology and technique has been perfected for the IUI, it is rare to see the use of the intracervical insemination. However, there are a few reasons for why it is still done today.

FACT

ICI has about a 2 percent conception rate for couples with fertility problems. This low rate leads most practitioners to do the slightly more invasive intrauterine inseminations.

The intracervical insemination is frequently done when the only problem is with sperm delivery—for example, if you were using donor sperm because your partner had a vasectomy—and you have no known fertility problems of your own.

The procedure is done after you have detected the LH surge during your cycle. You then contact the office and schedule the time for your insemination. You may also need to schedule a time for the semen sample delivery if you are not using donor sperm.

When Is IUI Indicated?

Insemination is the placement of sperm directly in or near your uterus in an attempt to help you conceive. Insemination is a minor fertility treatment designed to help overcome a few issues surrounding conception.

FACT

Insemination can be used even with various other methods of sperm retrieval. It is not necessary for your partner to masturbate—other forms of collection, like electroejaculation, can be used instead.

It can be used if you suffer from issues of sperm quality or quantity. Insemination is also used as a treatment for problems with cervical mucous, such as mucous that doesn't carry the sperm well through to the uterus. If your partner has erectile dysfunction or is for some reason unable to ejaculate inside of your vagina, insemination can also be helpful.

Insemination can also be done for the couple using donor sperm, because of an issue with the sperm, or because the woman does not have a male partner. This form of treatment is also appropriate for lesbian couples trying to get pregnant.

The intrauterine insemination is a great tool for you if you suffer from cervical stenosis. This can help bypass your cervical issues altogether and increase your pregnancy rates. The IUI is therefore a great alternative to the other treatments for cervical stenosis.

Meds or No Meds?

Insemination or artificial insemination is one of the few fertility treatments that can be used without medications. The decision on whether or not to use medications with your insemination can be based on many factors. Ultimately you, your partner, and your practitioners will have to make the decision as to what will work best for your situation.

Your diagnosis is probably the biggest criterion as to whether or not ovulation-inducing medications are used in conjunction with your insemination. If you suffer from undiagnosed infertility, it may be advised that you attempt a couple of inseminations, cervical or uterine, without medications. This can save you the expense of the medications and the required monitoring.

Natural (Unmedicated) Cycle

If all of your testing has been found to be normal and you ovulate regularly, having an insemination after a natural cycle may be a good option for you. Basically, you would check at home for your LH surge by using an ovulation predictor kit and call the doctor's office once you get your surge. The staff can then help you schedule your IUIs.

After three or four cycles of insemination only, it may be advised that you attempt to combine the insemination with oral medications to help ensure that you are ovulating. Taking medications such as Clomid and Serophene (clomiphene citrate) for a few days during your cycle helps accomplish this. The goals of these medications are not to create a huge number of follicles, but rather to produce one really good follicle for release and conception.

If you have tried clomiphene citrate-type medications for several cycles unsuccessfully, you may try injectable medications like Follistim, Gonal-F, or Repronex. These medications require more monitoring to ensure that you are not producing a dangerous number of follicles. This protocol is sometimes referred to as "superovulation," or "ovulation induction."

FACT

If you are having difficulty detecting your surge, check in with your doctor's office. They can usually help you monitor for your ovulation by having you periodically come in for bloodwork and/or ultrasounds.

Ovulation Induction

If you have not gotten pregnant after several attempts to conceive using more standard protocols of ovulation induction, it may be time to try using injectable medications in conjunction with insemination. This includes the use of medication to increase the number of follicles available to be fertilized at the time of your insemination.

ESSENTIAL

Many women are very nervous the first time that they perform their injection. But don't worry! It's very difficult to screw up and will get so much easier as time goes on. Make sure to ask all of your questions to the nurse teaching you how to do the injection, no matter how silly they may seem. They are more than willing to sit with you until you are comfortable.

While the actual manner of the collecting of sperm and insemination will remain the same, what changes are the protocols leading up to the insemination. Instead of doing your regular monitoring for ovulation, you will be placed on a regimen of medications to completely control ovulation, carefully controlled by your reproductive specialist.

How Ovulation Induction Works

You will be monitored via ultrasound during the medication period to check on the number and size of follicles that you are producing. You will also have blood drawn to determine if your hormone levels are adequate to help sustain the follicles and eventually a pregnancy. Using the information from the blood work and the ultrasounds, your physician will monitor and adjust the amount of medications you are taking.

Once your doctor determines that you have the appropriate number of mature follicles, you will inject a dose of hCG to simulate the LH surge, begin the final maturation of the eggs, and initiate ovulation. Then you will schedule your insemination. Typically, only intrauterine inseminations (IUI) are done for superovulation.

Collecting and Washing Your Partner's Sperm

There are plenty of jokes surrounding the process of collecting semen. The fact remains though that it is not a laughing matter; it is simply a fact of life. There is little, if anything, romantic about the process of collecting semen to be taken in for testing, insemination, or any of the other processes that are done with sperm. It can be very difficult for your partner to do.

It is recommended that your partner abstain from ejaculating for forty-eight to seventy-two hours prior to the collection of the semen for your insemination. This will ensure the highest quality and quantity sperm available.

Standard Collection

Typically what happens is that the man is given a specimen container, usually a sterile cup with a lid on it. The cup is marked with his name or patient ID number so that specimens are not confused in the laboratory. He is then taken to the collection room.

Collection rooms vary widely from fertility center to fertility center. Some fertility centers have comfortable chairs, erotic magazines, or videos for your partner to use to help him achieve erection, arousal, and ejaculation. You may or may not be able to stay with your partner during the collection process.

Some centers do not have specific collection rooms. They may use bathrooms as their collection rooms, and they may not have any "reading" material to help your partner with arousal. He may also choose to bring erotic materials from home.

ALERT

If you are able to stay with your partner, you are welcome to help him masturbate, though it is not recommended that you perform oral sex. Remember that the bacterial count is higher in your mouth than anywhere else in your body. In other words, spit harms sperm.

There are a few centers that allow the semen sample to be taken via a special condom. This can be much easier to obtain and it allows you to do the collecting at home; the sample is then required to be in the office within about thirty to sixty minutes. Be sure to ask if this is an option for your therapy.

Washing the Sperm

Once a semen sample is obtained from your partner, it will likely undergo a form of sperm washing in addition to sperm count and motility testing. Sperm washing is designed to remove the seminal fluid, which can be irritating to the uterus during insemination. It also removes dead sperm and other unnecessary cells. This is all in an attempt to increase the total number of motile sperm and your chances for pregnancy.

The procedure that is used will depend on the facility that you have chosen and perhaps medical factors in your case. Timing may also influence the decision to choose one method over another. Depending upon which method of sperm washing is chosen, it can take from one to three hours to complete.

Sometimes a centrifuge is used to wash sperm. A centrifuge spins the semen sample, which is mixed with a nutrient medium to aid in the washing process and separate the heavier and lighter fluids. The heavier layer at the bottom will contain the sperm-rich portion, which is removed from the centrifuge. The process is repeated several times to ensure that you are taking only the highest-quality sperm.

The sperm swim up technique is another technique used in sperm washing. Your partner's semen sample is layered with a washing medium on top. The best, most motile sperm will swim up to the top layer. This layer is then removed to be used for the insemination.

FACT

It is now believed that, by using sperm-washing techniques, we can allow men who are HIV positive to father healthy children. Since the HIV virus is found in the semen and not the individual sperm, it should be possible to use the sperm and not the semen to impregnate his partner without the risk of passing along HIV. This is used in conjunction with insemination or IVF procedures.

Which form of washing or what procedures are done after the collection takes place will depend on your fertility clinic. Be sure to ask if you have any questions or concerns before you begin treatment. You may also wind up doing several cycles, no two of which are alike.

Preparing for Your IUI

You will follow a fairly simple process if you choose to do intrauterine insemination. You will be monitoring your body for ovulation, either at home or at your clinic. When you are about to ovulate, the staff will tell you what further instructions you need. This will likely be a time for your partner's sperm sample to be given. You will be asked to come in a bit after your partner has made his donation of sperm. If you are taking medication, you will be instructed when to return to the office for your insemination based on your monitoring results.

The insemination usually takes place within the doctor's office or the fertility clinic. It does not require anesthesia. IUI is a fairly easy process that involves the placing of washed sperm into your uterus. Your partner will either bring in the sperm from home or produce it in the office. Once given to the lab, the andrologist will wash and prepare the sperm for your insemination. This process can take up to thirty to forty-five minutes, depending on the volume of patients within the lab. Make sure to clarify with your clinic about whether you should arrive with your partner and wait for the sperm to be washed, or if you can come back to the clinic at a later time in the day when you won't have to wait.

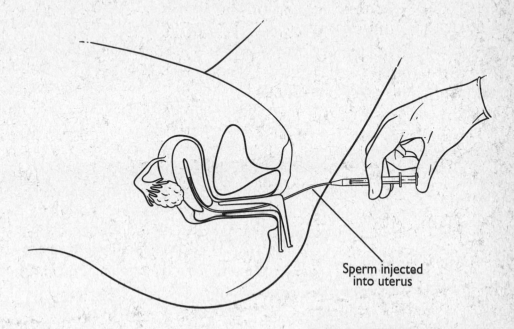

Sperm injected into uterus

Intrauterine insemination

Most women describe the feeling of the insemination to be that of a regular pap smear. After the washed sperm is placed inside the uterus, you will then lie on the examination table for about fifteen to twenty minutes to prevent any possible seeping of the sperm and its medium from the uterus. This is done largely as a comfort measure, as the cervix closes back down after the catheter is removed.

QUESTION

Why do I feel moist afterwards, if it's not sperm leaking?
The moisture you feel could be from cervical mucous being released by the procedure. Remember the procedure is timed so that it's done right around the time of ovulation, when increased mucous is often noted.

Once the sperm is ready to be inseminated, you will be escorted to an exam room and given a gown to put on. You will be asked to lie back on the exam table and a speculum will be inserted into your vagina so the practitioner can see your cervix. The cervix will be cleaned and prepped with a mild solution. A very small catheter will then be placed through the cervix and into the uterus. Once in place, the sperm will be injected through the catheter.

Most women report only the discomfort of the speculum being inserted, though some women do complain of mild cramping when the catheter is actually being passed through the cervix. This pain is usually very mild and brief. Your doctor may be able to recommend a mild pain reliever before or after the procedure to help minimize any discomfort. Tylenol is usually okay, though make sure to check with your doctor before you take anything.

If you are having intracervical insemination, the nurse practitioner will place the washed sperm near or just inside the cervix for dispersal. Sometimes a device similar to a cervical cap or diaphragm is used to hold the semen sample next to the cervix. You will be asked to lie there for a few minutes. If a cap was used, it may stay in place for the remainder of the day, depending on your clinic's protocol.

After Your IUI

After the intrauterine insemination, you may feel some cramping. Talk to your doctor or nurse practitioner about medications to control or ease pain from cramping. This procedure is usually not a cause for bleeding. If you do experience some bleeding, though, you may wish to call your doctor to reassure yourself. Sometimes the cervix is very tender and any manipulation, no matter how slight, can cause bleeding.

Generally, there are no restrictions on what you can do following the insemination. In fact, your practitioner might encourage you to have intercourse after the intrauterine insemination, just to cover all your bases. There is no real need to take it easy, but if you feel the need to refrain from aerobics or heavy lifting, you may do so. There is no indication that decreasing activity increases the chances of conception.

The doctor may recommend that you take hormone supplements, namely progesterone, to help boost your levels. This can help your body stay in a state that is ready for pregnancy. Finally, you will be instructed when to come back for your pregnancy test, or you may be told to call when you get or miss your period.

CHAPTER 13

In Vitro Fertilization

In vitro fertilization, or IVF, is one of the more invasive forms of infertility treatment; though for many couples it offers the greatest chance for success. If IVF is in your game plan, understanding the basics can make the process a little bit easier. Read on for the essential information you need before starting IVF.

What Is IVF?

Literally translated, "in vitro" means "in the glass" and refers to a procedure done in the lab. When combined with fertilization, as in "in vitro fertilization," it means that the fertilization of an egg with a sperm cell is done outside of the body and in the laboratory. And that is exactly what IVF is. Your ovaries are stimulated to produce many eggs, which are then surgically removed. They are then combined in the lab with your partners sperm so that fertilization will take place. The resulting embryos are allowed to develop for a few days and a select number are then transferred back into your uterus.

FACT

In vitro fertilization is used in fewer than 5 percent of all couples needing the aid of specialized fertility treatments and technologies, according to the American Society of Reproductive Medicine.

IVF was first used in England in the late 1970s. The first "test tube" baby, Louise Brown, was born in England in 1978. This launched a revolution in assisted reproductive technologies, making it possible for more families to conceive than before. Since 1981, in the United States, hundreds of thousands of babies have been born using IVF.

IVF Success Rates

IVF is used in cases that need extreme assistance in getting pregnant. This type of treatment is appropriate for you if:

- You have not conceived using other infertility treatments.
- You have tubal damage or scarring.
- You have missing Fallopian tubes.
- Your partner suffers from a low quality or quantity of sperm.
- You have unexplained infertility.

The success rates for IVF will vary from fertility clinic to fertility clinic. Overall, the American Society for Reproductive Medicine says that success rates are at about 22.8 percent for using in vitro fertilization, which is about the same rate for a fertile couple in any given month. This number is an average of all of the fertility centers participating in the Society for Assisted Reproductive Technology (SART) reporting.

It is important to note that the range of success for IVF varies widely. Usual quotes on the success rates are about 25–35 percent, though they can be between 0–70 percent. The range depends on a lot of different factors. Some variations are physical—like the reason for your infertility, your hormonal response to medication, and your anatomy. Other reasons for the dramatic differences in success rates depend on the fertility clinic and physician, their knowledge base, and their skill set.

Deciding on IVF

Making the decision to proceed with IVF should not be taken lightly. You should make sure that your calendar is clear for the weeks while you are cycling and that you have the time necessary to dedicate to your care. Anticipate being available for frequent monitoring, and you may need to be out of work at the last minute for your egg retrieval and embryo transfer. It can help if you prepare for these absences in advance; that way you are not as stressed out as if you were in the middle of a big project with an impending deadline.

Make sure that you have all of your medication and have cleared up any insurance issues in advance. Again, knowing that you have everything in order will eliminate some of your stress. Being prepared for the commitment it requires will make the process significantly easier on you in the long run.

Medications

You will need to take a number of medications while going through an IVF cycle. Don't worry though; your doctor or nurse will thoroughly explain your protocol and how and when you take each of the prescribed medications. It is important to take each of them exactly as prescribed by your doctor; not taking certain medications exactly when instructed can potentially ruin your cycle. Don't hesitate to ask any questions you may have; the staff will gladly clear up any confusion you have to ensure that your cycle goes smoothly.

Controlled Ovarian Hyperstimulation (COH)

You will likely need to take a combination of medications to both stimulate your ovaries and suppress your natural hormones. These medications are very tightly controlled to maximize your response while ensuring that you do not get sick. This is why you'll need to be monitored so frequently and why your medication will be adjusted frequently as well.

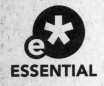

ESSENTIAL

Check out these helpful video guides to administering your medications: *www.ferringfertility.com/medications/trainingguide.asp* and *www.fertilitylifelines.com/resources/medicationguide.jsp*. The makers of Follistim and Antagon also have video guides on their website, *www.follistim.com/consumer/index.asp*, but you will need to navigate to the specific medication to find the instructional video.

Which suppressive medication you are prescribed depends on your age and diagnosis. Lupron (leuprolide), Cetrotide, and Antagon (Ganirelix) are common choices. You may also need to take a month or two of birth control prior to starting your IVF cycle. Your doctor will make the best decision possible using her clinical judgment.

Once your period starts and your cycle is ready to begin, you'll begin taking your ovarian stimulation, a combination of FSH and LH in the form of injectable synthetic hormones. Brands of these hormones include:

- Bravelle
- Follistim
- Gonal-F
- Menopur
- Repronex
- Pergonal

The purpose of these medications is to help the ovaries produce lots of eggs instead of the usual one. Keep in mind that your doctor will have her own protocols and will tell you exactly how to take the medication. You will take the stimulation medication for approximately ten to twelve days and will likely be in for blood and ultrasound monitoring every morning. Once your follicles are ready, after about ten to fourteen days on average on the medication, you will take a final injection of hCG that will trigger the final maturation of the eggs and prepare them for retrieval.

Hormonal Supplements

Once your eggs are retrieved, usually around thirty-six hours after your final hCG injection, you will need to start a new regimen of progesterone and estrogen supplements to strengthen your uterine lining and prepare your body for the embryo transfer. There are many different forms of progesterone. The most commonly prescribed are vaginal inserts or suppositories, and the dreaded progesterone in oil intramuscular injection. Sometimes, you may be asked to take a combination of both forms of progesterone, again depending on your clinic's policies.

ALERT

Make sure to ask how your progesterone should be stored, as it varies depending on the form. For example, the injectable progesterone in oil should be stored in a warm dry place, due to the potential of the oil congealing in the cold. On the other hand, the progesterone vaginal suppositories could melt if left out of the fridge.

You may also be asked to take an estrogen supplement to boost your estrogen level. This can take the form of either a pill or a transdermal patch, where the estrogen is absorbed through the skin. Remember, progesterone and estrogen are both the major hormones of pregnancy, which is why your doctor will want to make sure that you have as much hormonal support as possible.

Finally, depending on your clinic's policy, you will most likely need to take your antibiotic and Medrol, usually started around the time of your retrieval. These medications will help boost your chances of implantation.

Egg Retrieval

The egg retrieval, a surgical procedure to remove your eggs from the ovaries, is one of the most anxiety-provoking parts of undergoing IVF. This is particularly true if you've never had surgery before, but rest assured, the procedure is brief and relatively safe. Most clinics will have an anesthesiologist on site that will give you medication to help you relax or even fall asleep. The retrieval itself is only about twenty to thirty minutes long and recovery is usually pretty easy.

Preparing for Surgery

Once the doctor has instructed you to take your final injection of hCG, she will likely give you your preoperative instructions as well. If you will be sleeping during the procedure, you will be asked to refrain from eating or drinking for about eight to ten hours before the procedure. You should wear comfortable clothing and leave all jewelry at home. You might want to consider wearing your glasses that day, if you ordinarily wear contact lenses. Finally, they will give you a time to arrive at the clinic for you procedure. Try to be on time; likely there will be a lot to do to prepare before the surgery.

Make sure to ask about arrangements for your partner to produce his sperm—will he produce at home or at the clinic? Will you need to be with him when he produces? Is there anything you need to do for him to produce at home, i.e., pick up a sterile container? Discussing all of this beforehand ensures that everything will go smoothly on retrieval day.

What to Expect

When you arrive at the clinic, a staff member will escort you to the area where you will be prepped for surgery. You will be given a gown to put on and asked to remove all other clothing, including your underwear. If you are bringing sperm from home or need to be with your partner to produce his sperm, make sure to let the staff know ahead of time. Likely, you will not feel up to participating in his sperm production after the retrieval.

You will meet with both a nurse and the anesthesiologist prior to your procedure. They will both ask you questions about your medical history, allergies, medications you are taking, and other pertinent medical information. Quite likely, they will be asking you similar, if not the same questions.

This is not to annoy you, or because they aren't communicating with each other. Rather it is to make sure that they each have the most accurate information possible. The anesthesiologist will also need to start an IV so he can give you medications throughout the procedure.

ESSENTIAL

If you are nervous about becoming nauseous from the anesthesia, tell the anesthesiologist beforehand. They can pretreat you with anti-nausea medicine before you wake up. The anesthesiologist will also monitor you very closely to make sure that you are not nauseous after the procedure.

You will be escorted to the procedure room and placed into position. Your legs may be placed into the stirrups before you actually go to sleep. Don't worry though, the staff will make every effort to respect your privacy. The embryologist will also meet with you, either in the procedure room or before you go in, in order to identify you and make sure that the eggs are labeled appropriately once they are retrieved.

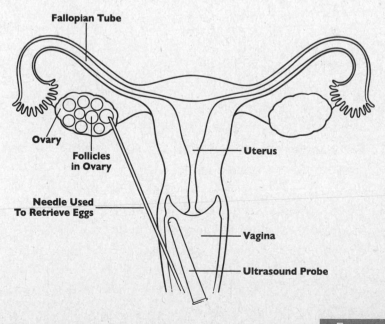

Egg retrieval

Once the procedure room and embryology staff is ready, you will be given medication through your IV to help you sleep or relax. Your doctor will then clean your vagina and cervix and insert the transvaginal ultrasound probe into your vagina. The probe has a needle attached to it. As the doctor is looking at the follicles on the ultrasound screen, he will use the needle to puncture the ovary through the vaginal wall and aspirate all of the fluid from the follicle. That fluid will go to the lab for analysis. Once all of the follicles have been drained, you will be woken up and sent to the recovery room. Most women experience a little cramping after the procedure, which is easily treated by Tylenol as necessary. Once you have fully come out of the anesthesia, you will be given your discharge instructions and discharged home to recover the rest of the day.

Recovery

Recovery after egg retrieval is generally pretty easy. You may have some light bleeding or cramping following the procedure, both of which are entirely normal. You'll want to take it easy the day of your retrieval, but pending your doctor's approval, should be able to go back to work the next day.

Your discharge instructions should include your new medication regimen and any restrictions that you need to follow until your pregnancy test. This may or may not include bathing (don't worry, showering is fine; you just want to avoid sitting in the water), intercourse, and any other activities your doctor wants you to avoid.

Though rare, it is possible to have complications after your procedure. Keep an eye out for any of these symptoms and make sure to let your doctor know if you have any of them:

- Severe pain or cramping that worsens over time
- Extreme lower abdominal bloating
- Fever
- Difficulty urinating
- A lot of sudden weight gain
- Feeling faint or dizzy

If you are not able to get in touch with your physician and are concerned about worsening symptoms after your retrieval, don't hesitate to go to the emergency room. You are always better off getting checked out, just in case.

In the Lab

Once your eggs have been retrieved, they will be given to a trained embryologist who will analyze and count them. By this point, they should also have your partner's sperm, which will then be placed in a Petri dish with your eggs. The dishes will be placed in the incubator overnight and allowed to fertilize. The following day, the embryologist will check the dish to see how many of your eggs actually fertilize to become embryos.

The Role of the Lab

The embryology team is wholly responsible for your embryos at this time. The embryos will be periodically checked to determine how well they are developing and will be assigned a grade to reflect that. This information of course will be given your doctor.

FACT

It's not abnormal for less than 100 percent of the eggs to fertilize and become good embryos. This can happen because of several reasons, including the maturity of the eggs, and the quality of the sperm may inhibit fertilization. Sometimes the resulting embryos have a genetic defect that prevents them from further development.

Finally, as the embryos are growing, they will need to be placed in special cultures to ensure that their environment is as similar to that of your Fallopian tubes and uterus as possible.

Are My Embryos Safe?

Rest assured. While every now and again, the story of a mistake makes the news, this is an extremely rare occurrence. The laboratory has a detailed and rigid plan in place for labeling and handling your embryos. In addition, the FDA and Department of Health have set specific guidelines when it comes to how your embryos are managed. Your lab must be periodically inspected by these organizations to ensure that they are complying with the state and federal guidelines. If the lab is found to be deficient, they risk losing their license.

Embryo Transfer

On either the third or fifth day after your retrieval, you will be instructed to come back into the office for your embryo transfer. Which day your transfer is depends on a number of factors that your doctor and embryologist will look at along with your medical history to determine which day is better for you.

On day five after your retrieval, your embryos should have progressed to the blastocyst stage. If your embryos are able to reach that point for transfer, it's generally better because that is the stage that embryos are in when they reach the uterus after fertilizing "the natural" way in the body. This is not always possible, however, depending on how the embryos have developed and your center's policies. Some clinics perform a majority of their transfers on day three; others will be more aggressive in extending embryos toward day five. Whichever day your transfer is, the procedure will be the same.

What to Expect

The procedure is very simple and is similar to having an insemination or pap smear. It's not painful and won't take very long at all. Many clinics will prescribe Valium for you to take approximately thirty minutes before your scheduled embryo transfer. Yes, it will help your anxiety, but this isn't the reason why you're taking it. The Valium is also a smooth muscle relaxant, which means it will help the muscles in your uterus avoid contracting when the catheter is placed through the cervix.

Once you have changed into a gown and have been prepped by a nurse, your doctor will come in and discuss the quality and number of your embryos with you. Quite likely, he'll make recommendations about how many and which embryos to transfer. He will notify the laboratory staff, who will also double check your identity and the number of embryos that are being transferred.

Once the embryos are ready to be transferred, you will be asked to lie back on the exam table and put your legs in the stirrups. A speculum will be inserted into your vagina and the doctor will clean your cervix. While all of this is happening, a sonographer will be looking at your uterus using an abdominal ultrasound. A special catheter will be placed through the cervix and into the uterus. It will then be advanced to the measurement that was taken when you had the special water sonogram before starting your IVF cycle.

The doctor will check the ultrasound to make sure that the catheter is in the correct place, then slowly load the embryos through the catheter and into your uterus. After it is removed, the catheter will be examined under the microscope to ensure that none of your embryos are left in it. Once the all clear is given, the speculum will be removed. You will likely be asked to remain in this position (though covered up) for a short period of time, usually around thirty minutes, and then allowed to head home.

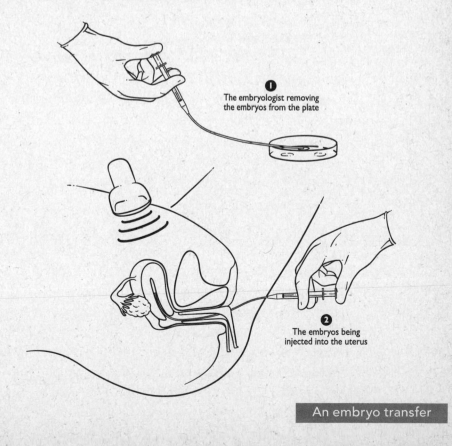

❶ The embryologist removing the embryos from the plate

❷ The embryos being injected into the uterus

An embryo transfer

After Your Embryo Transfer

Most doctors will ask that you remain on bed rest for one to three days after your transfer to keep your uterus as relaxed and calm as possible. This is thought to facilitate implantation of the embryos into the uterine wall. After your period of bed rest is over, you may be asked to modify your activity and rest as much as possible until your pregnancy test. You should be given detailed instructions about what to avoid and what medications to take after your transfer. You will continue taking the progesterone and estrogen supplements until you know the results of your pregnancy test, but the doctor may need to alter your regimen depending on your hormone levels.

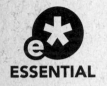

ESSENTIAL

You may feel fluid dripping out after the transfer, but this is just the fluid that was used to clean your cervix. Your embryos will not fall out once you stand up or go to the bathroom. They are safe and sound in your uterus and no amount of activity, even straining to go to the bathroom, can push them out.

Finally, you will be given a date to come back for your pregnancy test. You may be tempted to cheat and take a home pregnancy test earlier then your scheduled date, but don't forget that the hCG you took to prepare you for your egg retrieval is the same hCG that is detected by urine pregnancy tests. You will get a false positive if you test too early!

Assisted Reproductive Technologies (ART)

The beauty of fertility treatments is that the technology is evolving every day. New techniques are being developed to help patients overcome challenges to their fertility that doctors fifty years ago didn't even know existed. Many of these techniques take place in the lab and certainly aren't appropriate for every couple. Your reproductive endocrinologist should let you know which, if any, are in your plan. Many of them do cost extra and may not be covered by insurance. You'll want to investigate this early in the process so you don't get a surprise bill at the end of your cycle.

Intracytoplasmic Sperm Injection, or ICSI

For a long time there was little help available if your partner suffered from oligospermia or other conditions that result in very small numbers of sperm or damaged sperm. Without this sperm, the only treatment readily available was the use of donor sperm. This meant that there was no way for you to have a biological child that was also your partner's biological child. Fortunately, the ICSI procedure now makes it possible to overcome the problems of low sperm count.

FACT

The pregnancy rate using intracytoplasmic sperm injection (ICSI) is about 30 percent. This is a consistent rate for a typical IVF cycle. The difference is that these pregnancies are occurring where they previously never would have been possible without the ICSI technology.

Intracytoplasmic sperm injection (ICSI, pronounced "Ick-see") is a procedure in which a single sperm is used to fertilize a single egg. The procedure is done for each egg available after an egg retrieval. The retrieval of the sperm can typically be done under local anesthesia if the specimen can't be obtained by normal collection methods.

To begin the ICSI procedure, you will first enter an IVF cycle. You will be placed on medications that will cause you to begin to produce several eggs at once. As these eggs mature, you will go in for a retrieval of the eggs. During or just before the retrieval, your partner will have his sperm removed via fine needle aspiration through the testicle, by testicular biopsy, or by regular semen collection. The method used to retrieve his sperm will depend upon his diagnosis.

One single sperm is then placed inside a very small glass needle. Using magnification, the egg is visualized and the wall of that egg is penetrated using the glass needle. The sperm is then released into the egg's cytoplasm. This is repeated until either all of the eggs are used or all of the available sperm are used.

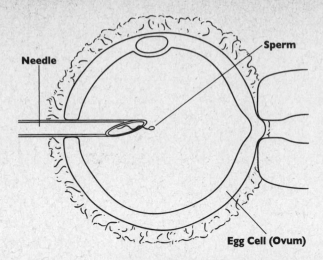

Needle

Sperm

Egg Cell (Ovum)

An intracytoplasmic sperm injection (ICSI)

Once the egg is fertilized, it is allowed to continue growing for between two and five days. At this point the egg is transferred back into your uterus using the thin catheter. This is exactly like the regular IVF cycle at this point.

QUESTION

Should we have ICSI even without sperm count issues?
Probably not. Using ICSI for cases other than those for male factor infertility issues and egg penetration issues hasn't been shown to improve pregnancy rates. Since it will add to the cost of your bill, it may be something better left out if it's not something you absolutely need.

The good news about ICSI is that fertilization is now possible with even a "weaker," less capable sperm. This is one of the best aspects of ICSI for the couples that need this type of technology.

Assisted Hatching

Another technology that may be able to help you conceive is called "assisted hatching." This can be used if your egg quality is low or there are problems with cellular division of the egg. Not all fertility clinics offer this technology.

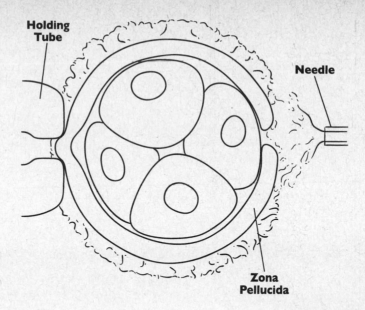

Assisted hatching

With assisted hatching, the egg is fertilized and allowed to develop as it normally would be in IVF. Once you are ready to have the embryos transferred, a hollow tube is used to deliver an acid solution to create a small hole in the shell or zona pellucida; the egg is then transferred shortly thereafter. The hole allows the embryo to hatch out of the zona pellucida, a process that must happen in order for the embryo to implant in the uterus. Some clinics use a weak laser beam to weaken the zona instead of the acid solution. Which technique is used will depend on your clinic and the qualifications of the embryologist.

Cryopreservation

The use of frozen embryos is another area where the technology is growing by leaps and bounds. Typically, in an IVF cycle, the fertilized eggs are used immediately. But there are also reasons that you might choose to freeze the embryos produced for later use.

The freezing of embryos is done for a variety of reasons. It may be done because your doctors have returned as many embryos to your uterus as possible (a number which is determined by many factors) and you have "extra" embryos remaining. You will pay about $500 to $2,000 a year to have the embryos frozen and stored to be available at a later date to be used by you for another pregnancy. In that case, the next time around you could skip the phase of ovarian stimulation in an IVF cycle and simply prepare the uterus for the transfer or return.

You might choose to use the frozen embryo program if you are about to undergo medical treatment for something like cancer that could potentially damage your reproductive system or ovaries. This allows you the option to have your own biological children at a later date when your treatment is completed and you are ready.

While the rates of pregnancy using frozen embryos are slightly less than those of using "fresh" embryos, the benefits are great. You will find that it is a lot less expensive and medically draining to do a frozen cycle. The need for preparation is much less and there is no need for the stimulation or egg retrieval phases of the cycle. This is a huge benefit for many families.

While the whole in vitro fertilization process is long and involved, the changing technology can offer hope to many families who previously could not have children even when you have had previously untreatable problems like severe male factor infertility. Though this technology offers new hope, it is not without pain and side effects and can lead to pregnancy or failure. The emotional aspects should also be considered when considering such an invasive and expensive procedure.

CHAPTER 14

More Assisted Reproductive Technologies

Assisted reproductive technologies (ART) are the big guns of infertility treatment. From test tube babies to tiny glass needles with a single sperm to analyzing a single cell in the embryo to determine the healthiest one, these are the technologies that are reserved for the most difficult cases and causes of infertility. While the success rates vary widely and may seem low, they are amazing successes for those who are involved in this ever-expanding field.

Gamete Intra-Fallopian Transfer (GIFT)

This treatment is very rarely done anymore and has been replaced almost entirely by IVF. There are still some women for whom this type of treatment might be appropriate. If you are staunchly opposed to IVF, perhaps for religious or moral objections pertaining to the potential destruction of embryos, GIFT might be more acceptable because fertilized embryos are not being destroyed. It may also be beneficial when the transfer of the embryos through your cervix is not possible.

A woman's eggs are prepared similarly to IVF when using GIFT. As the eggs are removed during the retrieval, the sperm is mixed with the retrieved eggs and immediately placed back inside the Fallopian tube. There is no waiting to see if fertilization occurs. You must also have at least one open tube in order to be eligible for this procedure.

There are several disadvantages to having GIFT. First, this procedure must be done laparoscopically, which is a more involved surgery. You will need general anesthesia and will have three small incisions made in your lower abdomen; this of course intensifies your recovery period. Also, your doctor has no way of telling which eggs will fertilize when he places them in your Fallopian tube. He has less control over the quality of the eggs he is transferring.

Success rates vary according to the program, but are usually comparable to those for IVF.

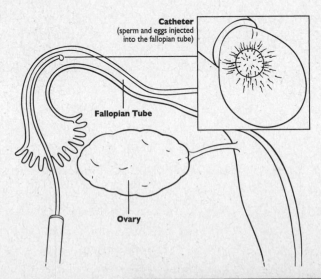

A gamete intra-fallopian transfer (GIFT)

Zygote Intra-Fallopian Transfer (ZIFT)

Another treatment used is called zygote intra-Fallopian transfer (ZIFT). A zygote is a fertilized egg that is at an earlier stage than an embryo. As the name suggests, your zygotes are transferred directly to the Fallopian tube rather than the uterus, on the premise that the embryos placed into the tubal environment may result in higher pregnancy rates. The chemical environment in the Fallopian tube is very different from the environment of the uterus. This procedure cannot be done if the woman does not have at least one open Fallopian tube.

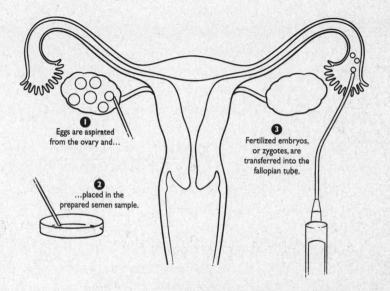

❶ Eggs are aspirated from the ovary and…

❷ …placed in the prepared semen sample.

❸ Fertilized embryos, or zygotes, are transferred into the fallopian tube.

A zygote intra-fallopian transfer (ZIFT)

Again, this procedure is very similar to IVF. Your ovaries will be stimulated with medications so that lots of eggs are released. Once they are mature, your eggs will be retrieved and fertilized exactly as in IVF. The big difference between ZIFT and IVF is that the resulting zygotes will be placed into the Fallopian tube, instead of the uterus. Also, the zygotes are transferred significantly earlier in the process, only a day or two after fertilization, so there is less time for the embryos to develop before selecting the best ones. ZIFT must be done under general anesthesia and is a more involved procedure.

You may hear ZIFT also referred to as tubal embryo transfer, or TET. Both procedures are very rarely done these days, despite some centers reporting higher pregnancy rates. The higher rates may not be because ZIFT is a better procedure; it may simply reflect poor transcervical transfer skills of the physician. Many physicians are also reluctant to use this procedure because of the need for laparoscopic surgery.

Not many centers routinely perform ZIFT or GIFT anymore. Check with the clinic before your first appointment to make sure that they offer these services if this is something that you're interested in.

Preimplantation Genetic Diagnosis (PGD)

Whereas some couples used to be counseled to avoid having children because of the risk of certain genetic diseases, technology has advanced to the point where embryos can be created, biopsied, and then only the healthy ones transferred. This has gone a long way toward preventing genetic diseases in couples who are known to carry the genes for them. For example, if you and your partner both carry the genes for cystic fibrosis, you have a one in four chance of passing it along to your children. Doing PGD eliminates that risk because you can select and transfer only genetically healthy embryos.

When you make the decision to proceed with PGD, you'll go through the entire IVF procedure: medications, egg retrieval, and fertilization in the lab. However, instead of preparing your embryos to be transferred on the third day after your retrieval, a specially trained embryologist will biopsy each of the embryos by removing one cell from each embryo. These cells will be sent to a specialized lab where their chromosomes will be analyzed. Your clinic will get a report within a day or two, informing your doctor which embryos are normal and which ones are abnormal. Your doctor can then make sure that she transfers chromosomally healthy embryos.

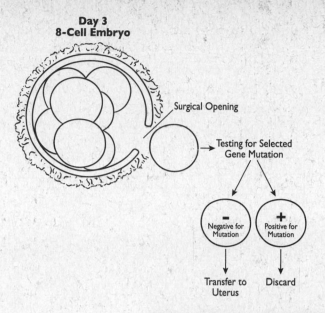

**Day 3
8-Cell Embryo**

Surgical Opening

Testing for Selected
Gene Mutation

−
Negative for
Mutation

+
Positive for
Mutation

Transfer to
Uterus

Discard

A preimplantation genetic diagnosis

There are two types of PGD: one where you screen for a specific genetic disease, and one where you screen for an abnormal number of chromosomes, also known as aneuploidy. Down's syndrome is one example of a disease caused by aneuploidy; a child affected by Down's syndrome has three copies of the twenty-first chromosome.

PGD for a Specific Genetic Disorder

If you are having PGD done to prevent a specific disease like cystic fibrosis, you and your partner will need to have blood or cheek swabs done first so that the lab performing the analysis can create probes that will precisely locate the mutation. It's important to know that this process might take up to several months, before you even start the IVF cycle. Once the probes have been completed, you'll be notified so that you can begin treatment with your clinic. Couples who have suffered multiple miscarriages for unknown reasons may benefit from preimplantation genetic diagnosis (PGD) to screen for genetic abnormalities that can't be otherwise diagnosed. If it is in fact a genetic abnormality, this can usually be corrected by transferring the healthy embryos.

PGD for Aneuploidy

If you have had multiple miscarriages or are older in age, your doctor may recommend that you have PGD to screen for aneuploidy. This may potentially diagnose a genetic cause to your pregnancy losses and can even prevent another one. Older women in particular are more likely to have genetically abnormal embryos result from the use of their own eggs, so having this type of analysis will help the doctor pick the healthiest embryos to transfer and increase your chance of pregnancy.

Other Reasons for PGD

Some couples are now electing to undergo PGD in order to select a particular characteristic for their child, like the gender or tissue antigen type. The antigen type, also known as HLA typing, is sometimes used to create a child who would be a good match to donate an organ for a sick family member. There has been some controversy regarding the ethics of this type of analysis, and as a result, some clinics only offer this service on a very limited basis, and many not at all. You should check with the clinic before you make an appointment.

FACT

Some clinics will only perform gender selection for cases of family balancing; where a family, for example, has many boys and now wants to have a girl. Others will not do gender selection at all because of the associated controversy.

If you choose to have PGD for gender selection, there are some questions you may want to talk about with your partner before proceeding.

1. What if the only genetically healthy embryos are the wrong gender?
2. Would we consider transferring embryos that are the wrong gender anyway?
3. How will we handle healthy embryos that are male if we want female, or female if we want a male? Discard, donate to another couple, or donate to research?

Cost

PGD can be quite expensive, depending on whether you have insurance coverage for the procedure. It is very likely, however, that your policy will not include coverage for this type of procedure because many insurance companies still consider it to be experimental. In addition to paying for the actual testing of the embryos, you'll need to pay for the biopsy procedure and to ship the embryos to the lab. Total cost can range from $6,000 to $10,000 or even more depending on your clinic, the lab they use, and the type of analysis you are having performed. This cost is in addition to the costs associated with the IVF procedure.

Sometimes, you may be able to petition your insurance carrier if the PGD needs to be done for medical reasons. The process can be quite involved and take a great deal of time, and still doesn't guarantee that you will be covered. But if finances are a major part of your concern, it may be worth trying anyway. Enlist the financial expert at your clinic; she may have some advice or experience in this area.

If you are having PGD for gender selection, tissue typing, or aneuploidy screening, there isn't much chance that your policy will cover the analysis, but you may be able to have part of the IVF procedure covered.

Mini IVF

Mini IVF is also known as micro IVF or minimal stimulation IVF and is very similar to the regular process of IVF. You will still take medications to stimulate your ovaries and to prevent ovulation from happening. Your eggs will be retrieved when ready, fertilization will occur in the lab, and healthy embryos will be transferred after three to five days. The main difference between mini IVF and conventional IVF is the number of eggs and embryos that the doctor and embryologist are working with—fewer with mini IVF than with the standard procedure. Whereas with regular IVF it's not uncommon to have ten to twelve eggs retrieved, mini IVF typically produces only three to four.

Advantages of Mini IVF

There are many advantages to using mini IVF. Cost is usually the most noticeable difference. A regular cycle of IVF without any insurance coverage at all can reach upwards of $15,000. A cycle of mini IVF is usually around $5,000 to $7,000. That's less than half the price!

You are also taking significantly less medication with mini IVF. Because the goal is to produce only a few high quality eggs, less medication is required to get you there. This is advantageous for several reasons; the cost of your medication is much less and your risk of ovarian hyperstimulation syndrome (OHSS), one of the primary complications of IVF, is also lower.

Disadvantages of Mini IVF

However, there are some cons to using this procedure. Because so few embryos are produced, it is highly unlikely that you will have extra embryos to freeze at the end of your cycle. This may not seem like a big deal if you only want one child, but think about what it will mean if the procedure doesn't work the first time. Thawing and transferring frozen embryos is significantly less money than both traditional and mini IVF.

FACT

Studies evaluating the success rates for couples undergoing mini IVF are not yet clear, with some centers reporting a wide range of pregnancy rates. Some centers show 20 percent, while others are claiming up to a 50 percent success.

A lot of couples don't like to talk about their IVF cycle failing, but unfortunately it is a fact of infertility treatment. There are lucky couples where it happens for them the first time, and there are couples that go through three, four, or even five cycles before they become pregnant. Doing multiple cycles of mini IVF may add to up to more money in the long run if the first few cycles don't work.

You also run the risk of having none of your eggs fertilize; this is not abnormal. This won't be a big deal if you have ten to twelve eggs because you still have a good number that will, but if you only had three eggs retrieved and two of them don't fertilize, that leaves only one to transfer. It's even possible to not have any of the eggs fertilize, leaving you with nothing to transfer and the whole cycle having been for naught.

Gamete Preservation

A relatively new area of fertility treatment is the preservation of your eggs and sperm for use later on. Many single women are opting to freeze their eggs to use later when they are ready to have children. This technology is also giving young men and women with cancer the ability to freeze their eggs and sperm for once their chemo treatment is over. This is especially important because chemo can cause infertility, as it often destroys the reproductive tissue. If a young cancer patient has their gametes frozen prior to beginning the cancer treatment, they may still have the ability to have children afterwards.

Cancer

Cancer of the female reproductive organs (the uterus, ovaries, and cervix) can potentially cause fertility problems. The medications and treatments used to help fight and cure your cancers can also wreak havoc on your uterus and ovaries. While on chemotherapy you might find that your periods stop completely. Sometimes this cessation of menstruation is permanent and lasts past your cancer treatments.

Infertility can also be a major issue for your partner if he has previously been treated for cancer. Many chemotherapy agents are known to halt or permanently alter sperm production.

FACT

World-renowned cyclist Lance Armstrong is a very notable voice for banking sperm prior to chemotherapy. He had banked his sperm for future use and used the stored sperm after he married former wife Kristin, with a combination of ICSI and IVF, for two pregnancies and three children! Read more about their story at *www.laf.org*.

If you have been diagnosed with cancer and wish to help preserve your fertility, be sure to discuss this with your oncologist and a fertility specialist. If your oncologist clears you to delay treatment for a month or so, you may be able to try to help preserve your fertility; this area is being heavily studied and new advances are being made all the time. One example might be to do a cycle of stimulation and have your eggs retrieved, fertilized, and frozen to be thawed for implantation at a later date. A man can easily plan ahead and make deposits at a sperm bank prior to beginning treatment for cancer.

Whatever your options, make sure to notify the fertility clinic that time is of the utmost importance because you need to begin cancer treatments right away. They should be able to accommodate you, but if not, try another office until you can find one that can.

Age

As more and more women are choosing to delay getting married and having children, they are becoming more aware that their "clock is ticking," so to speak. Many women are turning to fertility treatment to freeze their eggs to be used later on, when they are in a committed relationship or ready to have children.

While embryos and sperm cells freeze fairly well, unfertilized eggs are much more difficult. This is because they are the largest cells in the human body and contain the most amount of water. As the water within the cell freezes, it forms ice crystals, whose jagged edges could destroy the egg. In order to effectively freeze an egg, the embryologist must remove the water and replace it with a fluid that will not form these crystals when frozen.

ESSENTIAL

Frozen eggs have a lower thaw survival rate; only about 60–70 percent in women up to age thirty-eight. Therefore, some clinics may recommend that, depending on the number of eggs you produce, you undergo a couple of cycles in order to maximize the number of eggs you are able to freeze.

In order to freeze eggs, you will need to take gonadotropins to stimulate your ovaries, then have the eggs retrieved and frozen. Once they are ready to be used, the embryologist will thaw them and fertilize them with either your partner's sperm or the sperm from an anonymous donor. Your transfer will be a couple of days later.

Frozen Embryo Transfer

Most physicians will not transfer more than two or three embryos at a time, so what happens to the other embryos that are not transferred? Well, most labs will give you the option to freeze any excess, healthy embryos that are formed during your cycle. Doing so adds an additional fee and usually a yearly storage fee to your growing bill, but choosing to freeze your embryos can help you in the long run.

Having your embryos thawed out and transferred is considerably cheaper than a second fresh cycle, usually around $3,000. Storage fees can range from $500 to $1,500 per year. Sometimes this is covered by your insurance, sometimes only a portion of the cost is, and sometimes it isn't at all.

Process

Healthy looking embryos can be frozen on day three or day five after your retrieval, depending on when the embryologist and your doctor thinks is the optimal time. Currently, there are two methods that are being used to cryopreserve embryos: the traditional slow freeze method and a new ultrarapid method also called vitrification. More studies are needed to determine which process produces the best freeze and thaw survival rates.

ALERT

Make sure to check on your clinic's requirement for freezing excess embryos. Do they freeze all of the extra embryos, or do they have strict criteria for which embryos they choose to freeze? The more selective they are about freezing embryos, the more likely it is that the embryos will survive both the freezing and thawing process.

When you are ready to use your embryos, the doctor will prescribe estrogen supplements in order to prepare your uterine lining for the transfer. You will need to be monitored periodically to make sure that your lining is developing appropriately. The doctor may also prescribe Lupron to prevent ovulation, because once you ovulate, your hormone levels will change in a way that is unfavorable to the development of your uterine lining. Once your lining is ready, you will stop taking the Lupron, and add in the progesterone supplements. Your embryos will be thawed and transferred into your uterus.

Success Rates

The pregnancy rates after frozen embryo transfer are traditionally lower as compared to after a fresh IVF cycle. However, a lot of this depends on your clinic's criteria at selecting embryos for transfer, the skill level of the embryologist doing the freezing and thawing, and his experience with frozen embryos. You can check out the SART statistics for a clinic's frozen embryo cycles *www.sart.org/find_frm.html*.

Complications

There is always a risk that the embryo(s) will not survive the freezing and thawing process. If your clinic is freezing anything that is left over after your cycle as compared to having strict criteria for which embryos to freeze, it is more likely that some of the embryos they are freezing will not be great quality and therefore, less likely to survive.

Ethical Debates

It's quite amazing how far reproductive technology has progressed within the last twenty to twenty-five years. Scientists have developed a number of treatments to help couples that previously would not have been able to have children do just that.

However, you may find yourself struggling with ethical issues you never dreamed of when faced with the decision to use advanced techniques to help you achieve a pregnancy. Most likely your entire life you envisioned simply getting pregnant like everyone else does and spent little time, if any, addressing the potential quandaries of new technologies in the field of reproduction. You are not alone.

It is nearly impossible to turn on the television without hearing about the latest advances in technology surrounding the infertility field. Between all the legal battles about what is wrong and what is right rest your own opinions. What is important in this decision is that you, your partner, and anyone else that you feel the need to consult are appropriately pleased with your decision. You may choose to seek spiritual or religious guidance concerning the decision to use advanced procedures to help you get pregnant. Talk to your doctor about how to educate your clergy or spiritual advisor on the aspects of the fertility treatments you are considering. This can help you set your mind at ease so you can proceed as you see fit.

CHAPTER 15

Using Donated Sperm

In certain cases, the doctor may find that your partner does not produce a sufficient amount of quality sperm to warrant treatment using it. In this case, the use of donated sperm may be recommended to give you the best shot at pregnancy. In other cases, single women or lesbian couples may need to use donated sperm in order to have children. Whatever the reason, there are many things to think about before deciding on a sperm donor. Read on for more information.

Deciding on Using Donor Sperm

Sperm donation can be used for a variety of issues. You might choose to use donor sperm if your partner has problems with sperm production or mobility. This can also be useful if your partner does not have testicles, or if his testicles do not function properly. Many women may even choose to use sperm donors because they do not have a male partner.

Once you select a donor, check with the lab at your clinic to see what type and how many vials of sperm they'll need. Donated sperm comes in two forms: washed (IUI ready) and unwashed (ICI ready).

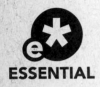

ESSENTIAL

Make sure to buy extra sperm for later use. That way if the cycle doesn't work, you'll have plenty to work with for subsequent cycles. And if you do become pregnant, you can use the sperm later on to have a second child. An added benefit is that your children will be genetically full siblings.

You'll need two vials per cycle. You may only need one vial if the sperm is to be used for IVF, but should get a second one as backup. Just in case the thawed sperm is inadequate on the day of the egg retrieval, there is another one available. If your lab doesn't have a back up sample and an insufficient amount of sperm, the cycle might be lost.

Male Factor

A couple may need to use a sperm donor in the rare circumstances where the male partner does not produce any or enough good quality sperm. Unless your partner doesn't have testicles or produce any sperm at all, the urologist your partner is working with will exhaust every possible treatment option with which you are comfortable. This may include medication or even surgery. In cases where the outcome of surgery is uncertain, it's strongly recommended that you buy donor sperm as back-up, in case the urologist is unable to find any sperm at all. If you and your partner are not okay with using donor sperm, even as a back-up, you may need to discard your eggs or consider freezing them for the future. Some men may choose to defer surgery and move straight to using donor sperm, and that's okay. Both you and your partner need to be on board with whatever treatment you use.

In cases where male factor infertility is the only issue affecting a couple's ability to conceive and donor sperm is the preferred treatment, you will probably start with donor insemination. You will undergo an insemination cycle either with or without medication, and then have the donated sperm inseminated, instead of your partner's. This is usually the least invasive option, and the one that your reproductive endocrinologist will likely start with.

Single Women and Lesbian Couples

It's actually relatively simple for single women and lesbian couples to have their own biological children; this is now made possible with the use of donated sperm. Whether you are in a lesbian relationship and want to start a family or are a single woman who is ready to have children even though you aren't married, you have several options for treatment.

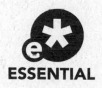

ESSENTIAL

If you choose an anonymous donor, make sure to purchase at least two vials of sperm for each cycle. You can purchase them all ahead of time, say six or eight vials, or you can purchase them each time you are about to cycle. Be aware though, that the sperm bank may run out of sperm from your donor.

You will have a full workup to make sure that there are no underlying fertility problems that could affect your treatment. Once you select a donor, you can proceed with whatever treatment your doctor recommends for you; be it insemination with or without medications, or even IVF.

Deciding Between Known and Anonymous Donors

Making the decision between a known and anonymous sperm donor is a challenging decision and one that should not be considered lightly. There are many factors that a couple or a woman should think about when making the decision.

Doing the Research

The first thing you need to do is your homework. Even if you're leaning one way or the other, it can't hurt to gather all the necessary information. Peruse the donor catalogs at a few clinics and see if anyone catches your eye. Call a few of the clinics and find out their requirements for known donor testing. Contact a qualified attorney and get information about your state's third-party reproduction laws. Also, don't forget to make an appointment with the counselor or psychologist at your fertility clinic. She can offer valuable insight that may be helpful when it comes to making the decision.

If your family or friends know that you will be using a sperm donor, it can't hurt to get someone else's opinion, too. After all, who else knows you (and your potential donor) well enough to help you decide?

Talking to Your Partner and Family

You should also consider the feelings of your partner. Will he feel jealous or resentful if he knows the donor? Will those feelings damage her relationship with the donor? Or would he prefer that his brother or very best friend in the whole world be the biological father, instead of an anonymous man?

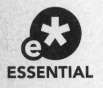

ESSENTIAL

Some lesbian couples elect to use a relative of the partner who will not be carrying the pregnancy or contributing her egg. This is a great way to pass on both families' genetic information into the child.

You don't have another partner to consider if you are a single woman, but you do have the rest of your family and possibly, his. If you think that choosing someone you know will create controversy or conflict within your family, you may want to think about using an anonymous donor to save both you and your child from lasting resentment.

Sperm Donation and Your Relationship

It may be easy to feel like it is your fault or your partner's fault. But imagine if the tables were turned and the conditions reversed. . . . How would you respond if you or your partner had fertility issues because of a previous battle with cancer? Would you blame your partner for having diabetes or asthma? Infertility is a disease that affects more than 15 percent of the child-bearing population. Keep that in mind before blaming anyone.

Men often experience a myriad of emotions when it comes to using donor sperm. These can include insecurity, guilt, anger, denial, embarrassment, and everything in between. He may be wondering how you feel about him now that he can't provide you with children, or if you will leave him. He may feel guilty at everything you have to go through just to have children. His feelings about the sperm source should be heavily considered when making the decision also.

If this comes as a bit of a shock, your partner may need some time to adjust to the fact that he will not have a biological child. He may want to get a second opinion or try aggressive forms of surgery to know that at least he's tried everything. On the other hand, he may be dead set against using donated sperm at all. If this is the case, you will need to discuss what your next steps will be.

Using a Known Donor

There are both positives and negatives to using a known sperm donor. When you know the donor, you know his personality, his family, and his medical history. Your child will also have the ability to know her biological father if she's interested later on. The cost is also probably less because you won't need to pay the donor for his sperm.

FACT

Some banks offer the option of a "willing to be known" donor, an anonymous donor who is open to the possibility of a meeting in the future. This is the best of both worlds: someone who is not involved in your daily life or your family, but who may be willing to meet at your or your child's request.

You should consider the disadvantages as well. If you are not planning on telling your child that she was the result of sperm donation, be aware that that kind of secret can be used in an argument later on. Whether or not it's intentional, the result is not the same. It's also possible that your donor could eventually try to sue for custody on the grounds that he is the biological father. Finally, the legal and counseling costs incurred could add up to be quite expensive.

Legal Issues

Before committing to using a known donor, make sure to consult with a reproductive attorney. Your fertility clinic can help direct you to someone who has experience in dealing with third-party reproduction. This is absolutely essential because not every state has laws that honor the arrangements between a couple (or woman) and her known sperm donor. If your contracts and the legal documents aren't in order, the donor can theoretically request adoption or even custody of your child, simply because he is the biological father.

Personal Issues

Think about how you'll feel if you run into or routinely see your donor. Imagine how he'll feel, when he looks at his child and knows that she is his biological child, too. How will your family react to the information that your child is not your partner's biological child but, for example, your brother-in-law's? Not all family members are so open, which can understandably create a great deal of conflict.

That being said, some families are completely encouraging of this type of arrangement and would bring a lot of positive support to everyone involved. The challenge is in knowing which type of family you have.

If the man you are thinking of asking to donate is married, this can create additional conflict as well. Will his wife support the donation and the fact that her husband has a genetic child outside of their marriage? Some clinics require that the donor's wife attend counseling appointments also, just to make sure that she is supportive of the situation.

ID Testing

If you are using donated sperm from a nonintimate (i.e., sexual) partner, federal regulations require that he undergo a rigorous series of tests to screen for infectious diseases. This will include blood testing, a physical exam, and an extensive interview to evaluate his sexual habits. Any high-risk behavior may be concerning, as it increases the risk of his contracting an infection that could be transmitted through his sperm. For this reason, only frozen sperm can be used, never fresh.

ALERT

Some clinics might waive the quarantine requirement when you use a known donor, but this is very strongly discouraged because of the risk of spreading a serious infection like HIV or hepatitis. Regardless of whether the quarantine was waived, you will only be able to use frozen sperm.

Once the man has been cleared to donate, his sperm will also be checked for infection and then frozen. It will remain in quarantine for six months. Because HIV and hepatitis can take a while before they show up in a person's blood, your donor and his sperm will need to be retested at the end of that six-month quarantine. This minimizes the chance that the donor had contracted a serious infection, but that it was too early for the blood testing to reveal it.

Some couples choose not to go this route, or it may not be feasible to wait for the six-month quarantine because of the female partner's age. Anonymous sperm that has been quarantined already and is immediately available may be a better choice.

Anonymous Sperm Donors

If you choose to use an anonymous donor, you will have a great deal of information at your disposal. Most banks will provide a catalogue of donors, so that you can look through and significantly narrow down the choices based on your (or you and your partner's) ethnicity and physical characteristics. Some ethnicities may be harder to find then others.

Finding and Selecting a Bank

There are a number of sperm banks that provide this service. Chances are good the one you choose will not be in your hometown, so a lot of your interaction with the bank staff will either be via e-mail or over the phone. Make sure that the bank you select has a license to do business in the state in which you live. Here are a couple of the larger, well known sperm banks:

California Cryobank
www.cryobank.com
(800) 231-3373

Fairfax Cryobank
www.fairfaxcryobank.com
(703) 698-3976

Xytex Corporation
www.xytex.com
(706) 733-0130

Idant Laboratories
www.idant.com
(212) 244-0555

Each facility will have their own policies when it comes to the amount of information they provide and the cost at which it comes. Some banks will give you basic information for a nominal fee, and then provide you the "deluxe package" for a higher fee. That level of information may or may not be important to you, but you should make sure that you are comfortable with what the bank will provide you. If you are interested in the "willing to be known" option, you'll also want to make sure that the bank offers this option.

How to Choose a Donor

Typically donors are bright, young, college men who are paid to donate their sperm. They too will undergo a number of tests to screen them for infectious diseases. Some banks may even require a personality test or IQ test, though not all of them do. Again, the frozen sperm will be quarantined before you are able to use it.

Depending on the bank you choose, you may be looking at pages and pages of sperm donors. How in the world do you choose one? Well, you'll want a donor that closely resembles you and your partner. Some factors to look at:

- Hair and eye color
- Skin tone
- Height and weight
- Ethnicity
- Religion
- Blood type
- Level of education
- Current occupation

Not all of these factors may be important to you. It may even be impossible to find a donor who matches you and your partner in each and every one of these characteristics. But you'll want to pick the most important ones to you and work from there. For example, maybe instead of only Italian donors, you'll consider Mediterranean men. Or include men with green eyes, instead of only blue. It can also be helpful to consider your family members when thinking about a donor. For example, if you have brown hair, but a lot of close family members are blonde, you might want to expand your search to include lighter haired donors.

Sibling Donor Registry

As the children of donor sperm and eggs have gotten older and started looking for their biological parent and other siblings, the need for a donor registry emerged. In 2000, the Donor Sibling Registry (DSR) was formed to help these children find half siblings from other donations and even the identity of their donor and his family. The registry also provides assistance in searching for your biological father and resources for donor sperm offspring.

You can also find an abundance of resources and studies on the site, all related to issues very specific to donor siblings. Remember that a lot of this is uncharted territory. Research has long shown the benefits of disclosing to your children that they were the result of donor sperm treatment, and this service now gives them the opportunity to find siblings and family members that they didn't know they had. It can provide closure to many of the questions that come up—about their identity, their other biological family, and medical/genetic history.

FACT

You can find the sibling donor registry online, at *www.donorsibling registry.com*. Registering costs $50 per year; all you need is the names of your clinic and sperm bank.

The good news amidst all of this is that the final decision rests with you and your family. No one but you and your partner need know what reproductive technologies you've used, even when they involve a highly trained team of specialists to pull off a pregnancy.

CHAPTER 16

Using Donated Eggs

One of the newer ideas in the area of reproductive technology is that of egg donation. This practice is becoming very popular for a variety of reasons, and the technology can now help women overcome fertility issues related to egg quality or quantity. The process of egg donation has not been without controversy, but this has not slowed down the use of this ever-broadening aid in the field of fertility.

When Is Using an Egg Donor Appropriate?

Egg donation is a relatively new technology in the field of infertility treatment. It affords new hope to previously infertile women who have poor egg quality or quantity. Egg donation involves the removal of eggs or oocytes from one woman (the egg donor or donor) and placing them into the uterus of another woman (the recipient). This can be beneficial for a variety of reasons.

Egg donation provides hope if you are suffering from premature ovarian failure, if you have had your ovaries removed, if you have been through menopause, or if you are unable to ovulate for any other reason. It can also be used if for some reason you cannot use your own eggs, as in the case of genetic problems or concerns.

Pregnancy rates with egg donation vary, but are much higher for many couples than doing IVF with their own eggs. This can be due to the factors that are causing your infertility, or simply the fact that the donors are typically younger and are more likely to have a higher degree of fertility. Always be sure to ask about the donor egg success rates of your particular fertility center before starting the process.

Preparing for Your Cycle

Once you've made the decision to proceed with egg donation, you'll need to do some research. There are many things that you'll need to consider before you are ready to select a donor. Using an egg donor is a very extensive process and very much more involved than using a sperm donor. Your donor will need to go through most of the IVF process: She'll take the injectable medications and go through the egg retrieval. That also means she'll be in for monitoring every morning, thus committing a great deal of time and energy to the process.

Cost

A single cycle of egg donation can easily run $15,000 to $30,000, depending on the type of cycle you are doing and if you need any additional treatments, like ICSI or cryopreservation. In addition to your medical costs, like screening, medication, and your embryo transfer, you'll also be paying for all of her expenses, including her medication, monitoring expenses, her egg retrieval, and screening. Most clinics also purchase a temporary health insurance policy for her so that any medical costs (related to potential complications from her cycle) incurred during the cycle are not passed on to her.

ALERT

Keep in mind that your insurance will not cover any of the expenses related to your donor. Your policy may cover your transfer, medications, and basic testing. You should follow up with your insurance policy to determine what, if anything, will be covered.

Finally, if you are using an anonymous donor, you will need to pay her compensation. This varies widely according to where you live and the standard rate in that area. It can range from $4,000 to $8,000 per cycle, or even higher. You should know that the American Society for Reproductive Medicine ethics committee guidelines state that "Total payments to donors in excess of $5,000 require justification and sums above $10,000 are not appropriate." There are many clinics and agencies that pay their donors above $5,000 based on the local "going rate," but you should be wary of any center that tries to charge you more than $10,000 for donor compensation.

Exclusive Cycles

Most clinics offer two types of cycles: shared and exclusive. Which one you choose will depend on you. If you are using a known donor, or sometimes even an agency donor depending on the policies of your clinic, you will need to have an exclusive cycle. When doing an exclusive cycle, all of the eggs retrieved from the donor will become yours.

The cost, of course, is much higher than when sharing the eggs, but you are much more likely to have frozen embryos at the end of your cycle, simply because you are likely going to receive more eggs. Having frozen embryos is beneficial because if it doesn't work, it will be much less expensive to do a frozen transfer than to do a second cycle. Also, if you do become pregnant and want to have more children, having those frozen embryos to use means that your children will be full genetic siblings.

Shared Cycles

The other type of cycle is a shared one. This happens when your donor is matched both with you and another recipient at the same time. All parties involved remain completely anonymous, meaning that you don't know anything about your donor or the other recipient and they don't know anything about you.

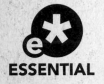

ESSENTIAL

Sharing a donor splits the donor's cost between the two recipients, making the cycle significantly cheaper and often more feasible for couples. Keep in mind though that you'll also be sharing the eggs retrieved from the donor.

All three of your menstrual cycles will be coordinated together and you will be dependent on each other as the cycle proceeds. This means that if your other recipient has, for example, a small ovarian cyst that requires waiting a month or two before cycling, you will need to wait too. It also means that they will wait for you if you need to delay cycling for a month.

The eggs retrieved from your donor will be split in half and distributed evenly between you and the other recipient. Some programs may have other policies in place for couples that share a donor, so make sure to ask. However, because you only receive a fraction of the eggs, you might not have embryos left over to freeze.

Using a Known Donor

Using a donor you know, or a known donor, is another popular option in the field of egg donation. You may have a friend or family member who is willing to donate her eggs to you. This is usually a great option for you if you have this available.

Using a known donor, and hence the eggs of someone you know, can give you many benefits. It allows you to be more genetically related to your baby (if your donor is your sister or other relative). It can remove some of the fear of the unknown out of the process. It also allows you to have contact with your egg donor.

While all of these points may be beneficial, they may also weigh heavily on your mind. You may wonder if the stress on the donor is too much. Perhaps you're worried about everything you are putting her through. It's best to be open and to discuss these issues with whomever you've chosen as your donor. This can prevent hurt feelings and feelings of frustration down the road.

Even when you are using a known donor, you will be asked to see the psychologist or mental health professional at your clinic. This meeting will usually include the donor as well as yourself, and may also include the partners of both you and your donor.

Who Should I Ask?

The woman you ask to donate her eggs must match the criteria set forth by your clinic. She should be in her twenties or early thirties, healthy, and, of course, not a blood relative to your partner. She shouldn't use drugs or smoke cigarettes (they can affect egg quality). Most importantly, her hormonal testing should indicate an adequate ovarian reserve.

How Do I Ask Her?

Now, let's say you have someone in mind to be an egg donor, but you don't know how to approach her about the issue. Look for signs that this person might be open to being a candidate and find a time to talk when neither of you will be interrupted. She may or may not know of your struggle to have a child. You might have to fill her in on the details.

Once you have told her of your fertility journey, explain to her the process of egg donation. Tell her that you would be honored if she would help you by being your egg donor; then tell her you want to give her space and time to think about the proposal. This is, after all, a huge decision. Explain that you have a host of people who would be willing to talk to her to get her more information if she needs it. Also assure her that your relationship will not be harmed if she chooses to decline being your egg donor.

Then back away and give her space. She may have questions you can't answer. She will possibly need to consult with other people before making her decision, like her husband or partner, her religious counsel, or her doctor or midwife.

When doing a donor cycle, sometimes you are able to get more eggs than you can use. These eggs belong to you. You will be able to attempt to save them for a later cycle and complete a frozen embryo transfer.

She may not agree to this proposal; this might be something that she cannot do for whatever reason. If this is the case you do need to respect her desire without letting it hurt your relationship.

Selecting an Anonymous Donor

Choosing a donor is a huge deal. The person that you and your partner choose will be the DNA behind your future baby. For some couples, they do not wish to know who this person is or much about her. This anonymity is very important to them.

Your fertility center may also participate in a program for donor recruitment. That means you are allowed to go out and place ads or otherwise solicit egg donors. A potential donor contacts the fertility clinic directly, so you avoid all contact with her, and her eggs are earmarked specifically for you if she is determined to be suitable.

You and your partner may prefer an unknown donor. This may be because you do not know anyone who would make a suitable donor for you, or it may be that you prefer not to know the donor. Either decision is perfectly appropriate. Having an anonymous donor is more common than a known donor in many areas. It also prevents you from having to explain your fertility issues to someone else, if you have chosen to keep your fertility problems a secret.

Your fertility clinic will have a protocol by which a donor is chosen for you. You will be asked to select criteria you wish to base your choice of egg donor on. This could be eye color, hair color, body build, ethnicity, religion, or any number of other factors. Some fertility clinics will offer you physical and educational sketches of potential donors. Some fertility centers may also ask you to send in a photograph. Ask your fertility treatment team or the donor egg coordinator what the actual process is for your center.

No matter how your donor is chosen for you, be sure that you are completely comfortable with the process. As you've read multiple times, this is a huge decision and not one that is made lightly. Talk to the donor egg coordinator at your fertility center about how the process is kept anonymous. This will help you if you fear finding out who the anonymous donor is for your cycle.

The cost of an unknown donor may be slightly higher per cycle than that of known donor. This is because there is usually some form of compensation offered to the donor for her time and trouble in this setting. There are agencies set up to do nothing but provide fertility clinics with egg donors. They are usually more expensive, but often do more extensive searching for the egg donors. This may reduce the wait you have for a donor.

Factors to Consider

Choosing an egg donor may seem very overwhelming, and a lot depends on the system your fertility clinic has in place. You will be given specific instructions and advice on picking a donor. Though the process varies a bit depending on which type of donor—known or unknown—you "choose to use."

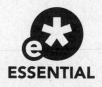

ESSENTIAL

Ask your fertility center about donor matching fees. Do they charge a fee to match you with an egg donor? If so, how much is it? What services are included in the fee? Is it refunded if they do not find a donor? Will it be waived if you find your own donor?

No matter what, when choosing a donor you are likely to have physical, mental, and emotional preferences. If there is something that you feel very strongly about, remember to talk to your egg donor or your fertility center's donor coordinator about your preferences. Here are some typical things that you may have a preference about in your egg donor:

- Age
- Religious background
- Ethnicity or cultural background
- Genetic issues
- Hair color
- Eye color
- Education level
- Hobbies
- Availability for a second donation
- Height
- Weight/body type

Factors used in selecting a donor like hobbies and educational background are not known to directly relate to what your future child will be like. However, they may be more comforting for you or for the potential donor.

Whomever you decide to use as you choose a donor is perfectly acceptable. Do not let the preferences of others influence you as you make your decision. This needs to be a 100 percent decision for you and your partner.

Screening the Donor

Most egg donors are between the ages of twenty-one and thirty-four. This is the current recommendation by the ASRM. Women over the age of thirty-four have an increased risk of genetic problems in pregnancy (for example, Down's syndrome) and a decline in natural fertility. Some fertility centers also require that the egg donor have proven fertility, meaning she has been successfully pregnant prior to her egg donation.

One of the first steps in selecting a woman as a donor is a psychological evaluation. The potential donor will usually have a one-on-one chat with a psychiatrist, psychologist, or social worker, depending on the fertility clinic. This professional is someone who is familiar with the special needs and issues surrounding egg donation.

Once the egg donor clears this stage, the physical exams begin. Some fertility centers choose to start with blood screening. The egg donor's blood will be tested for drug use, medications, diseases, and so forth, to ensure that the donor is in good health.

FACT

Most fertility centers will provide the donor with short-term health insurance to cover problems that arise from the donation. This fee is usually charged to the recipient. This prevents the recipient from suddenly having to pay out of pocket should some medical problem arise from the egg donor's harvest or treatment.

In addition to the blood work, the donor will undergo a complete physical exam. Some fertility centers allow this exam to be performed by the donor's own physician, while others choose to have the physical exam done by their office. This will include examining her reproductive tract and screening for reproductive health.

A detailed medical history is also taken at this time from the egg donor. Occasionally, she may be referred to a genetic specialist if there are questions and concerns about her genetic history.

Using an Egg Donor Agency

An alternative to having your clinic find your donor is to contact a private egg donor agency whose sole purpose is to recruit donors. Generally speaking, an agency has a greater selection of donors. Working with an agency to find a donor can also be a lot more expensive. In addition to paying the match fees, which are usually higher then what you'll pay at your doctor's office, you'll also pay travel fees for your donor and a companion. That includes airfare, hotel, and food expenses. The companion needs to be with her for after the egg retrieval, so she's not alone in case of complications.

If you are looking for someone with a very particular set of traits, and your clinic doesn't have anyone who fits that description, it may be beneficial to check out a couple of agencies to see if they have a donor that you might like. You do need to be careful though; if you select an agency donor, she must meet the criteria set forth by your clinic. Before agreeing to work with an agency, you should ask a lot of questions:

- What happens if the donor isn't accepted by my clinic for medical reasons? Can I get my deposit back?
- What happens if she begins taking medications and she doesn't respond well or is canceled because of a medical reason? Do we get a refund?
- Do you have any donors that are local to where I live?
- What kind of information can we get about her?
- What is your financial policy?
- What are my legal obligations?
- Have you worked with our clinic before?

You should get all of this in writing before you agree to use the agency. You can ask to see a copy of their contract and consult with an attorney before you sign any paperwork.

ALERT

You'll also want to make sure that the agency is licensed to work in the state where your clinic is. The clinic will need a copy of their license before working with them, otherwise they won't be able to do business with the agency.

Cycle Coordination

Once you have selected your egg donor—whether it is a known or anonymous donor—you will choose a time to synchronize your cycles. It is imperative that you both be hormonally regulated to the same cycle, using a variety of medications.

Synchronization is a very important step in the process of using donor eggs. This will ensure that your uterus is at the right phase to accept the eggs from the donor at the time they are ready. If this step is not done, or if it is done incorrectly, it can lead to an entire cycle being wasted.

What She Does

Your donor will begin oral contraceptives during her period. She will then be placed on a medication like Lupron to prevent her from ovulating too early. After the Lupron she will begin taking stimulants to induce ovulation. Remember, the goal is to get as many good-quality healthy eggs as possible in one retrieval. She will be monitored by blood work and ultrasound to choose the day to trigger her for release and retrieval.

What You Do

You will also be preparing your body during this process. You will not be taking stimulants to help you ovulate; instead you will have your ovulation suppressed during this cycle so that you do not spontaneously ovulate, usually by taking Lupron. You will be given estrogen supplements to help build a strong lining (endometrium) in your uterus.

QUESTION

Will I run into my donor at the fertility center?
Great care is taken during anonymous cycles to ensure that the egg donor and the recipient's partner are not in the fertility clinic where they are able to run into each other. Even if the donation is anonymous, and the two parties would have no reason to know one another, this is still very important to many couples.

Once the eggs are retrieved, they will be fertilized with your partner's sperm or donor sperm (whichever you have decided upon). The eggs will typically be incubated for several days before you will take part in the embryo transfer. Any remaining embryos that are not put back into your uterus are normally frozen and are yours to use at a later time.

Once the embryo transfer is done, you begin the two-week waiting period to see if the pregnancy takes hold. Waiting for the pregnancy test is difficult. You will be taking daily progesterone to supplement your body to support the pregnancy. This will continue until your reproductive specialist tells you to stop, usually until you are about twelve weeks pregnant.

Cycle synchronization is a vital element to your egg donation. Talk to your doctor or fertility team if you have any questions about how it will be done. This can be a very exciting time, but it can also be a time of worry. You have to leave the control of the stimulation medications to the egg donor that you may or may not have contact with. Take heart in the fact that many of the egg donors who are anonymous have done this before. The egg donor is also given all the tools she will need for a successful cycle.

CHAPTER 17

Using a Gestational Carrier or Surrogate

The legal case of Baby M catapulted the use of surrogacy as a means of becoming a parent into the spotlight. While most of the cases involving surrogates are not splashed all over the tabloids, using a surrogate involves a bit more than other forms of resolving fertility issues previously discussed. Surrogacy is definitely something that you and your partner must be willing to tackle head on.

A Gestational Carrier versus Surrogacy

People often interchange the terms gestational carrier and surrogate, thinking that they are the same thing. But they're not. There are some important differences and which one you need will depend on your individual medical situation.

Gestational Carrier

A gestational carrier is a woman who carries the pregnancy and has no genetic link to the child. Embryos are created through IVF from the couple's own eggs and sperm. The embryos are then transferred into the carrier's uterus. This is the treatment of choice for a woman who has her ovaries, but who is either has no uterus or whose uterus is unable to support a pregnancy. This can an ideal treatment for someone who is not healthy enough to carry a pregnancy or who has had a catastrophic event after her last pregnancy.

ALERT

All of these procedures can also be done with donated sperm if indicated. That circumstance could get kind of sticky, since neither partner would then have a genetic link to the child. This opens the possibility of the surrogate to request and win custody of the child, since she is the only genetic link to the child.

Surrogate

A surrogate is a woman who is carrying a pregnancy, but the embryos are created using the carrier's eggs and the male partner's sperm. So in essence, the surrogate is the biological mother of the resulting child, because her eggs contributed to half of the child's genetics. This can be accomplished with the use of insemination where the carrier is inseminated with the male partner's sperm. IVF can also be used in which the carrier undergoes the entire treatment, from ovarian stimulation to egg retrieval to embryo transfer. The partner's sperm would be used to fertilize the eggs in the lab.

This treatment is used either when the recipients are a homosexual male couple who would need an egg donor in addition to the carrier, or when the female partner also needs an egg donor and gestational carrier. This could be because she was born with the complete absence of her reproductive organs, or because she had them removed for a medical treatment.

Is Using a Carrier for Me?

The relationship between a recipient couple and their carrier or surrogate is a very special and unique one. It is a special situation that most people will not be able to understand, unless they've been through it themselves. You are essentially placing your trust, your money, and most importantly, your child, in another woman to nurture and protect. You will need to trust that she's taking care of herself and going to her prenatal visits. Before jumping into using a carrier or surrogate, make sure to carefully weigh the positives and negatives to determine if it's the right choice for you and your partner.

Advantages

First and foremost, using a carrier can give you and your partner the opportunity to have a child, using both of your genetics. This may not be possible otherwise. If you choose a carrier who is open to sharing the experience with you, you can still be involved in her pregnancy, her prenatal appointments, her ultrasound visits, and hopefully even the delivery. It can be helpful to decide on what type of relationship you want in her pregnancy, so that you can find a carrier who wants the same level of involvement.

Disadvantages

In addition to all of the typical IVF and pregnancy worries, you'll also likely have concerns about the legal status of your agreement. Using a paid gestational carrier or a surrogate is not legal in many states. This of course contributes to a great deal of complexity. Perhaps you had to keep your agreement with your carrier under the table, or you may worry that the formal contract you were able to draft won't hold up in the event that your carrier changes her mind.

There's also the possibility that the relationship between you and your carrier could sour. If you have been trying to get pregnant for a long time, you will likely be nervous throughout your carrier's pregnancy, and that could manifest in unrealistic expectations, like demanding that she not eat any artificial preservatives. Your carrier will most likely be more relaxed about the pregnancy then you will be, leading to possible conflicts.

Financial Issues

Working with a gestational carrier or surrogate can be prohibitively expensive, with total expenses ranging anywhere from $45,000 to over $100,000, depending on the clinic you are working with.

FACT

None of the costs related to your carrier's pregnancy will be covered by insurance. In fact, many policies have specific exclusion policies for women who became pregnant as a carrier or surrogate. This is why you need to cover all of those extra costs.

The reason that this is so costly is that you must be able to cover all of the expenses related to your carrier's pregnancy and the IVF cycle(s) needed to create the embryos. You might see fees for:

- Health insurance for the carrier
- Invasive procedures (including amniocentesis, selective reduction, etc.)
- Lost wages/housekeeping for bed rest
- Multi-fetal pregnancy
- C-section
- Life insurance
- Carrier fee
- Legal fees for both you and your carrier
- Miscellaneous expenses related to her medical care and doctor's appointments
- Travel expenses

As you can see, these fees add up quickly. Of course, all of these might not apply during your cycle, but even if everything goes perfectly, it will still be a costly venture.

Important Questions

There are some important issues you'll want to iron out as well. What happens if your carrier doesn't become pregnant after the first cycle? The second cycle? Will you get your money back, or will you be tied into using this carrier? Multiple cycles of IVF add up significantly. What happens if there is a late-term loss? Nobody likes to think about those things, but how the worst-case scenarios will be handled should be addressed ahead of time. That way, you aren't faced with a legal or financial fight in addition to dealing with your grief.

International Surrogacy

In an effort to minimize costs, some couples are opting to go overseas for their treatment. India, in particular, is a common destination for couples that bring their embryos to special clinics where they are transferred into the womb of one of their carriers. The cost varies by clinic but can be less than a third of the cost of using a gestational carrier in the United States.

This sounds great at first glance, but before you book your trip, you should think about a few of the downsides. There has been some ethical debate about paying these women significantly less than what they would be paid elsewhere. The opposing argument is that the money they make from one cycle could be more than they make in a year. That money makes it possible to provide food, clothing, and a better life for their family.

The other issue you'll want to think about is your child's citizenship. There have been cases where the intended parents had a lot of difficulty obtaining a visa to bring the child home and, in some cases, having their home government recognize the child as theirs. Make sure that you have spoken to an attorney about how to handle this situation and what your options are before committing to treatment.

Legal Issues

You will usually have a contract with the carrier that spells everything out in detail, not just finances. You may want to include issues like who can attend the birth or what, if any, contact she will get to have with the baby after birth.

You might spell out what happens in case the fertility procedure produces multiples. There are many legal issues to consider.

Remember that while you may be nervous about the process, most of the time everything goes very smoothly. Women choose to be surrogates because they are kind, generous people who wish to share with you the gift of parenthood. Talking to your partner or even the agency or support group can be a good way to work through any worries that you may have about using a carrier.

FACT

Reproductive attorneys are specially trained to interpret the tricky laws pertaining specifically to reproductive technologies. Other attorneys don't have the training necessary to handle such difficult legal situations. You can find a reproductive attorney at *www.theafa.org/ resources/lgbt_professional_network/all/category/attorney*.

The most important thing to know about using a carrier or surrogate is that not all states recognize the contract between a carrier and the prospective parents as valid. You will need to make sure that all of your "Is" are dotted, and "Ts" are crossed. Consulting with a reproductive attorney is a good place to start. She can give you all of the information about the laws in your state and will help you draft the necessary contracts to minimize the risk of legal complications.

Finding a Carrier

Finding a carrier you can trust and work with for the next year or so is one of the most important parts of the process. You must also consider the legalities in the state in which you live; there are many states where it is illegal to compensate a gestational carrier. This means you may need to use someone that you know instead of an agency surrogate. Many people will do this and arrange compensation under the table. Keep in mind before considering this that you have no legal recourse if something goes wrong.

Using a Known Carrier

Many couples will consider asking a very close family member or friend as their first choice. Quite often, that person has seen what that couple has gone through trying to have a baby and has either offered or will agree to help them. A clinic will usually only agree to use a known carrier if that person has been through the emotional and physical challenges of pregnancy and labor. She must know what to expect in terms of the pregnancy and what it will mean to hand the baby over at the end of it.

Your carrier must be in good health and able to carry a pregnancy. Her family must be supportive of her decision and help care for her throughout the process. In fact, both she and her husband (if she's married) will probably need to come to a meeting with the psychologist at your clinic before she can proceed. She will also need to be thoroughly screened for a number of infectious diseases, to minimize the risk of an infection being passed on to the baby.

Using an Agency to Find a Carrier

If legal in your state, it may be a better choice for you to use an agency-recruited carrier. Agency carriers have usually done this before and are experienced in the process. That can be reassuring, as they may be less likely to back out or change their minds.

FACT

Because carriers can live all over the country, it's important to ask where she lives before selecting someone. This is particularly important if you want to be involved in the pregnancy and want to go with her to her appointments. Obviously, if you want this type of relationship with her, she'll need to be somewhat close to where you live.

Depending on the agency's policy, the carrier has most likely been through a rigorous screening before being matched with you. This includes both medical and psychological testing to ensure that she is able to go through the pregnancy.

What Does Treatment Involve?

Treatment with a gestational carrier or surrogate is similar to standard IVF—it's just the players that change. Everybody involved in the process will need to be thoroughly screened for infectious diseases. This could include the intended parents, if they are contributing their eggs and/or sperm, the gestational carrier, and the egg donor, if one is used. In addition to the medical evaluation, all parties will need to participate in a psychological evaluation to make sure that they are fully prepared for the coming cycle. Once all the testing is complete and accepted, you'll be ready to proceed.

Treatment Using a Gestational Carrier

If you are using a gestational carrier, that is, you will still be contributing your eggs but just having another woman carry the pregnancy, you will need to undergo IVF. Your ovaries will be stimulated with a combination of follicle-stimulating hormone and luteinizing hormone, so that you produce many eggs. Those eggs will be retrieved and fertilized with your partner's sperm (or donated sperm if necessary) in the lab. The resulting embryos will be transferred into your carrier on the third or fifth day after the retrieval.

This can also be done using an egg donor in addition to the carrier. There are all sorts of reasons why a couple (or woman) may choose to use an egg donor separate from her carrier. Perhaps the woman she wants to donate her eggs isn't comfortable carrying the pregnancy. Or maybe it's the other way around; the woman who agreed to carry the pregnancy doesn't also want to be the biological mother of the child. Whatever the reason, the treatment is exactly the same, except that it is the egg donor who will be going through IVF to produce her eggs.

While you (or your donor) are taking your stimulation, your carrier will need to take a combination of estrogen and progesterone to prepare her uterine lining for the transfer. After the transfer, and if she is pregnant, she will continue taking those supplements to help support the pregnancy.

With a Surrogate

If you are choosing to use a surrogate, a woman who will both donate her eggs and carry the pregnancy, IVF isn't necessarily the treatment of choice. The doctor will likely first try several cycles of insemination where she will have your partner's sperm inseminated while she is ovulating. She can either monitor for her ovulation at home or through blood tests and ultrasounds. The doctor may even recommend low doses of ovarian stimulation to better her chances of becoming pregnant.

There is no field as ripe for debate and ethical consideration as that of reproduction. As it has been for years, who, why, and how you conceive is a highly debatable topic. Add a bit of science to the pot and the issues for debate are at even higher stakes.

Religiously speaking, issues concerning pregnancy and birth are always minefields. While some topics like sperm donation are for the most part readily accepted, there are some organized religions that still consider even this treatment to be unethical.

ESSENTIAL

It can be beneficial to consult your spiritual advisor as you are starting this journey toward parenthood. She may have very particular feelings about what can and shouldn't be done a part of your treatment. Understanding this beforehand can help define your boundaries as time goes on.

You and your partner should have a lengthy discussion about your beliefs and religious and ethical considerations before expanding into any territory that leaves either of you feeling uncomfortable. If the two of you can live with your decisions, do what you feel is right.

From the simple donation of a single cell to the adoption of a live infant, third-party pregnancy certainly has its share of medical, legal, and ethical debates. While the most important decisions should be made between you and your spouse, it is important to talk about your beliefs and how they might affect your child-to-be. Do the research and figure out if third-party reproduction is something that appeals to you on an emotional level, a financial level, or even an ethical level. Make the decision that is right for you and your family!

CHAPTER 18

Complementary Therapy

There has been a lot of focus recently on doing things as naturally as possible and on using alternative therapies as a means of treatment. Complementary medicine is a great way to boost your natural fertility and can sometimes even help make your infertility treatment more productive. Be wary of unrealistic claims though; if it seems too good to be true, it probably is. Read on for more information about the different alternative therapies and how to determine what's right for you.

Acupuncture

There have been quite a few studies that looked at the effectiveness of acupuncture in making IVF more likely to work. Some preliminary research has shown a very slight increase in pregnancy rates in women who underwent acupuncture with their IVF cycle as compared to women who did not. Much more research is needed before a definite link can be established between acupuncture and successful fertility treatment.

What Is Acupuncture?

Acupuncture uses small needles that are placed into various points in the body to regulate the way your body functions. Reproductive acupuncturists seek to manipulate your uterine lining and ovarian function in order to optimize your body for pregnancy. The belief is that regular treatment can help increase blood flow to the uterus and ovaries, which is known to help thicken and enrich the endometrium.

FACT

Sometimes your doctor will allow the acupuncturist to give you a treatment in the clinic before and/or after your embryo transfer or insemination. A treatment right at that crucial time can help direct blood flow to the uterus and encourage implantation. If not, make alternative arrangements with your acupuncturist.

You should start your acupuncture treatment at least a few weeks before you begin your fertility treatment, or before you begin trying to get pregnant. Your practitioner will put together a protocol for you, but treatment once a week is common. Whatever your treatment plan is, speak with her ahead of time so that you know what to expect throughout your cycle.

Who Can Benefit from Acupuncture?

Keep in mind that acupuncture will not treat major structural disorders like endometriosis or pelvic adhesions. Those are only treated by medical or surgical therapies. However, the acupuncture can help boost blood flow and healing, and might even be able to reduce your pain. Some women have reported a more regular menstrual cycle and less cramping. The good news is that acupuncture is not contraindicated for anybody, or any medical condition, and it certainly will not negatively impact your cycle.

Are There Risks?

Acupuncture does involve placing small needles all over the body. While the risk is small, the needles used can cause or even transmit infection if not disposed of in between patients. For that reason, you must make sure that your practitioner is at least licensed and board certified. There are many acupuncturists who choose to specialize in reproductive issues, and you should find someone who has experience in treating infertility. Check with your clinic to see if they have any recommendations. There may be someone they work with regularly.

Herbals

The use of herbal products has exploded in recent decades, so these therapies are readily available in most locations. Many people have returned to using herbs and herbal medications for a variety of reasons.

Using Caution

Some herbs are said to have properties that aid in conception. They may or may not help you in your quest to conceive.

ALERT

Many herbal products can interact with medications you are taking. Be sure to tell your practitioner about *any* herbal products that you are using, no matter what the purpose is for the herbal product. This can prevent potential complications for your health down the line.

Herbs and herbals are not held to the same high and strict standards of medications, so you should proceed with caution. The use of herbs should be discussed and carefully monitored by an herbal practitioner. Use your phone book or look online to find someone who specializes and has had advanced training in their use. Often health food stores will have contact information for these practitioners as well. By consulting someone who is trained in the use of herbal medications, you can be sure you're using the specific type and amount that is the best for you.

Meeting with an herbal practitioner is usually a good idea. This meeting will consist of a screening for health problems and discussion about your current condition, medications you are taking, and what you intend to achieve. The herbal practitioner can then help you find products that could assist you in conception.

Useful Herbs

Red clover is a plant that is said to aid in preparing the body for conception. It is usually recommended in tea form—the plant and capsule forms do not prepare the body in the same manner. This is used to help cleanse the uterus and reproductive tract. For fertility uses, the blossom of the red clover is usually prepared from dry form as an infusion or tea. Susun Weed, a well-known herbalist, recommends taking a cup of dried blossoms and steeping them in a quart of boiling water for at least four hours, but preferably overnight. You can drink this infusion, serving size one cup, up to four times a day. To make this infusion a bit tastier, try adding a teaspoon of dried peppermint. Remember, herbs are not a quick fix; they can take months to aid you on your road to conception.

Red raspberry leaf tea is also said to be a uterine tonic. This means that it can potentially tone your uterus for and during pregnancy. The belief is that if your uterus is "fit" then you are more likely to conceive. You can purchase premade teas and tea bags of red raspberry for this purpose. Or, you can make your own by boiling water and adding the leaves to steep for about an hour. Again, add some taste to this concoction by adding peppermint.

Herbs to Avoid

There is a list of things that should be completely avoided in the preconception period. Many of the herbs that are commonly used are known to cause late periods or have a history of being used to actually prevent conception. Here is a small list of some of the herbs to avoid while trying to get pregnant:

- St. John's Wort
- Dong Quai
- Wild carrot (Queen Anne's lace)
- Blessed thistle
- Parsley seeds
- Stinging nettle
- Dill seeds
- Wild yam
- Caraway seeds
- Oatstraw
- Celery seeds
- Pennyroyal
- Cumin seeds

Avoiding these herbs and products made with them is a good idea. When in doubt, ask your practitioner or herbalist about the safety of a particular herb.

Your Weight

More and more studies are showing how important it is to be at a healthy weight before you try to conceive. Being severely over- or underweight can affect the balance of hormones in the body because fat cells can produce estrogen. Too much fat, and your body has an abundance of estrogen. Too few fat cells, and your body can be missing vital supplies of estrogen. In either case, your fertility can or will be affected.

Make sure that you incorporate lots of fruits, vegetables, and whole grains into your diet. You should also take a multivitamin to guarantee that you are getting all of the essential vitamins and minerals that you need. Try incorporating a little extra activity into your life. Go for a walk each day, try some muscle building activities; even yoga has been shown to have a beneficial effect on your fertility, as you'll see later in this chapter.

Nobody has said that giving up the foods you love and adding in more exercise is easy or fun. And your doctor certainly isn't being mean when he tells you to lose weight. But if there's one thing that you can do to help boost your health and fertility, this could be it. Isn't it worth it to have a healthy pregnancy and baby?

ESSENTIAL

It may be tempting to go on a crash diet right before your cycle so that you can lose lots of weight somewhat quickly, but this is not a healthy thing to do. You're likely to put the weight back on, and possibly even more than what you lost.

Yoga

People have been practicing yoga for thousands of years. Advocates point to the many benefits that regular practice can have. This is a great way to help you deal with stress and find balance, strength, and even confidence. Physically, it can help build muscle and reduce tension, and some experts even say that working through certain positions can help boost your fertility!

Yoga for Fertility

Yoga will not cure the underlying cause for your infertility, especially conditions like endometriosis, pelvic adhesions or scar tissue, and uterine fibroids. However, when used in conjunction with traditional infertility treatment, it can help boost blood flow to the pelvis and reproductive organs.

FACT

It can be helpful to take a class with a certified yoga instructor. A great yoga instructor can really help you get started and give you further advice about positions that can boost your fertility. She'll also make sure that you are progressing through the poses appropriately.

Many women who perform yoga on a regular basis report feeling more connected to their body and more at peace emotionally. Yoga also enhances a feeling of well-being, which can carry over into the rest of your life, encouraging you to make healthier choices in your diet and activity.

Yoga Positions

The following positions have been shown to benefit your fertility. Try incorporating these poses into your regular practice.

Bridge Pose

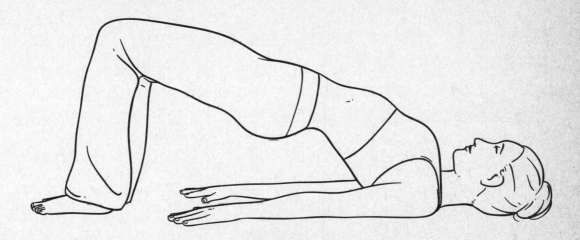

Setu Bandha Sarvangasana pose (Bridge pose)

Lie on your back with your knees bent and your heels as close to your buttocks as possible. You can place a small towel under your shoulders to support your neck. Gently lift your hips and buttocks until your thighs are nearly parallel with the floor. Keep your knees over your feet, but push them gently away, opening up your hips. Hold for thirty to sixty seconds and then slowly roll your spine back down into a lying down position. This pose works directly on the uterus and can help relax other reproductive organs in the pelvis and lower abdomen.

Legs Up the Wall Pose

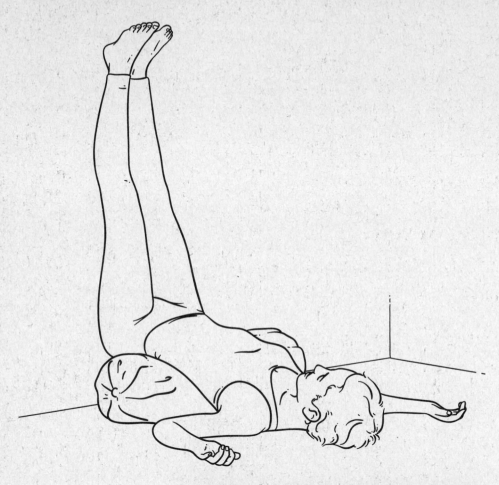

Viparita Karani Pose (Legs up the Wall pose)

Place a few folded towels about six inches from the wall. Sit on the edge of the support and in one swift motion, swing your legs up and against the wall. Your buttocks should shift off of the support and settle between the towel and the wall. You may need to experiment with your support (how high it is and how far from the wall it is) until you find what works for you. You can place a small rolled towel under your neck if it is more comfortable for you. Hold this pose for five to fifteen minutes. This pose can help relax your abdominal muscles and calm your mind.

Corpse Pose

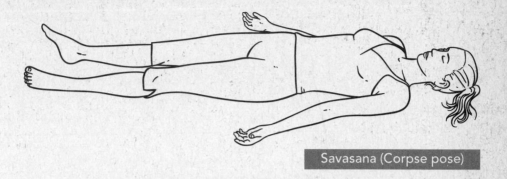

Savasana (Corpse pose)

Lie on your back with your legs and arms stretched out and equally distant from the center of the body. Keep your hands and feet soft, with the palms turned up and your feet falling to the side. You can place a small towel under your head and neck for extra support if you need. Try to relax every muscle and organ in your body and quiet the mind. Stay in this pose for about five minutes. To leave, slowly roll onto your right side and stay for a few breaths, then slowly sit up, dragging your head behind you. This pose calms the mind and can help reduce stress.

Bound Angle Pose

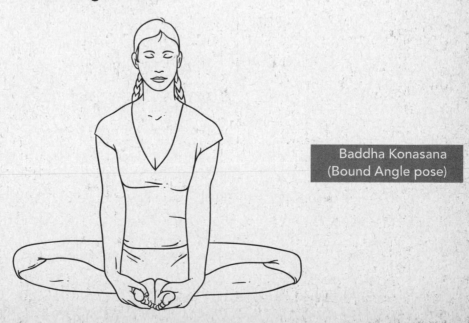

Baddha Konasana
(Bound Angle pose)

Sit on the floor or towel with your legs stretched out straight in front of you. Gently pull your heels in toward your groin as close as is comfortable for you. Hold your big toes with your first two fingers and thumb. Sit so that your perineum is parallel to the floor and lightly stretch the front of your body through the top of your chest. Open your thighs so your knees fall softly to the floor; never force them. Stay in this pose for one to five minutes. This pose stretches and strengthens the pelvis and reproductive organs in the lower abdomen. It also helps relieve depression and anxiety.

Supported Shoulderstand Pose

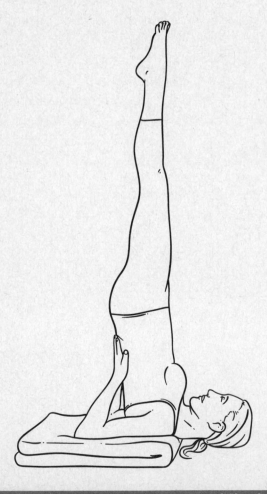

Salamba Sarvangasana (Supported Shoulderstand pose)

This is considered to be an intermediate to advanced pose and should only be attempted with an instructor who can help you get into the proper position. Fold two to three blankets and place them on the floor. Lie on your back so that your shoulders are supported on the blankets and your head is on the floor. Your legs should be stretched out. Gently bend your knees and roll your hips so that your knees come in toward your chest.

Because this pose can be tricky for a beginner, you should check out www.yogajournal.com/poses/480 for more information on getting in and out of this pose, especially if you are not used to regular yoga practice.

As you lift your pelvis off the floor, bend your elbows and turn your arms so that your hands can support your back. Keep your thumbs pointed toward your face. Your thighs should now be parallel to the floor with your knees bent and your feet hanging over your buttocks. Breathe in and push your heels toward the ceilings, then point your toes upwards. Stay in this pose for about thirty seconds, especially as a beginner. You can lengthen the amount of time you are in this pose as you become more experienced. This pose helps relax the abdominal organs and is especially helpful in treating infertility.

Relieving Your Stress

Stress can kill your fertility. Whether you are in the beginning of your journey toward parenthood, or have been trying for many years, finding ways to manage your stress is crucial to boosting your fertility. Stress isn't just bad for your emotional health, but can cause persistently elevated levels of other hormones, like cortisol and epinephrine, which may play a role. It's also thought that reducing your stress can help the uterus express proteins that are necessary for implantation.

Multiple studies have shown the benefits of stress reduction before and while trying for pregnancy. They've shown that couples are more likely to get pregnant when they are happy and relaxed and less likely when they are feeling anxious.

Stress While Undergoing Infertility Treatment

Infertility treatment is a stressful experience on its own. Unfamiliar procedures, nightly injections, possible surgery . . . all of these have the potential to induce a tremendous amount of stress on anyone. Many couples go into credit card debt, take out loans, or lose a big chunk of their savings, which can also contribute to a couple's stress. Add in the uncertainty of whether it will all work in the end, and no wonder that women report being extremely tense before and during treatment.

The tension that you are experiencing while undergoing infertility treatment is to be expected and completely normal, but it's important that you find ways to manage it as you move into treatment.

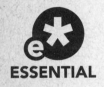

ESSENTIAL

If you're able, take a small vacation before you start so that you are in a calm and relaxed state of mind. It doesn't have to be an elaborate two-week extravaganza, but taking a long weekend to get away and reconnect with your partner is important.

Take advantage of your reproductive psychologist or social worker and solicit her advice for specific tips that she has found to be effective. It can also be helpful to delay cycling until work and your personal obligations have calmed down a bit. Make treatment your primary focus and make sure that you are able to dedicate the amount of time necessary. Facing treatment on top of your busy season at work can easily cause you to feel out of control.

Stress Reduction

Finding ways to manage your stress is an absolute must when trying to get pregnant. It is one of the best ways that you can increase your chances of getting pregnant, both naturally and with treatment. There are lots of things you can do to help cut down on your stress. First, reduce your unnecessary obligations. Don't feel like you have to take on extra projects or favors for others; learn the value of saying "no." A simple "I'm sorry, but it's really not a great time for me to ____" will usually get the point across.

It's very important to find time for yourself too. Schedule a workout, a movie with friends, or even a regular massage. Find something to look forward to, and schedule it regularly! After all, you'll want your body happy, calm, and relaxed for your pregnancy, right? Well, now is the time to start!

Evaluating the Effectiveness of Alternative Treatments

Spend some time on the Internet and you'll likely come across a multitude of ads and websites promising the next best herbal supplement or technique for guaranteeing a pregnancy. Unfortunately, there is nothing you can do that will guarantee that pregnancy will result. That bears repeating—there is nothing that you can do to guarantee that you will conceive. So, be wary of anyone who promises you otherwise. Yes, there are steps that you can take to help your body prepare for a pregnancy and increase your own natural fertility. But that is a very different claim than a guarantee of success.

When doing research online, make sure to check out reputable sites and sites that have been medically reviewed. Anybody can post anything online; it's not all accurate. Stick with well-known sites and sites that are in compliance with the Health on the Net Foundation's HONcode standard for trustworthy health information. In order to receive and maintain this designation, a website must demonstrate their commitment to publishing only medically accurate information. And as always, talk to your doctor or nurse before you try anything. Even all-natural and herbal supplements can be bad for pregnancy or your health, so you should double check before taking anything.

CHAPTER 19

Coping with Infertility

Dealing with infertility is a challenge. It's easy to get caught up in the doctor's appointments, monitoring visits, and nightly injections without taking too much time to deal with your emotional health. But this is such an important part of your treatment and if you don't find a way to find a positive support system, it can quickly sneak up on you and get overwhelming. Ahead, some tips!

Staying Sane

From playgrounds at the park to baby showers for your friends, there are probably babies everywhere you turn. When you are trying to have a baby of your own, it seems like everyone else is the world is either pregnant or already has a child. This can seem like a cruel twist of fate.

Your emotions may go back and forth wildly—both from hormones and just simply from the stress of what you're dealing with. You may find yourself feeling down or depressed. You may be angry at life or yourself or your doctor or your partner. You may be feeling guilty. These are all normal feelings. With the many mood swings that are possible, you may feel like you are going crazy.

FACT

Don't forget that you are taking medications that can increase moodiness. Some women have likened it to PMS times a thousand. Knowing this won't fix how you're feeling, but can help you feel better that you could be experiencing a side effect of your medication.

Keeping your sanity while in fertility treatments can be difficult at times. You are asked to balance work, testing, fertility treatments, appointments, and all for what? All for the chance to have a baby? It can simply seem overwhelming and unreal at times.

Finding a way to deal with these emotions is imperative. You need an outlet to help you vent and find something good to focus on in your life. You need something outside of the world of fertility. This may mean getting involved in a new hobby or finding a sport you enjoy. While it won't solve your problems, it can help you find the physical or mental release you need and a bit of escape as well.

Depression and Infertility

It's no wonder that so many women and couples who are going through infertility treatment suffer from some symptoms of depression. For a process that is so seemingly natural and easy, it can seem completely unfair to be facing so much needed help and assistance. You may compare yourself with other parents, wondering "why they could have children, but we couldn't." You can drive yourself crazy, questioning if it was the pot you smoked in college or the abortion you had in high school.

Symptoms of Depression

Symptoms of depression include difficulty eating or sleeping, having trouble concentrating, losing motivation, eating or sleeping too much, feelings of sadness and hopelessness, and becoming withdrawn from your family and friends. You may not even notice the symptoms until your partner or a friend points them out to you.

FACT

Check out this free screening tool online: *http://depression.about.com /cs/diagnosis/l/bldepscreenquiz.htm.* Answer the questions to see if you are possibly experiencing signs of depression. This tool is not meant to diagnose you as depressed, but can help encourage you to get help.

It is important to know that depression is a disease, a chemical imbalance of some important hormones in the brain. There should be no shame or embarrassment in asking for help if you need it. Talking out your feelings with an impartial person can really help you gain perspective and insight, and help you manage treatment just a bit easier.

Treatment for Depression

Treatment for depression varies widely among sufferers, depending on their life situation, the severity of their symptoms, and even the education of the counselors they see. Different therapists study different modalities of treatment, including behavioral, cognitive, or eclectic (a mix of a bunch of different types). Sometimes "talk therapy" is recommended, where you sit with a therapist and work out your emotions while talking with her.

If your symptoms are severe, your counselor may suggest medication and recommend that you see a psychiatrist. He will evaluate you and determine if medication is in fact appropriate for you. It is really important that you be upfront with your doctor about the fact that you are trying to get pregnant. Some medications cannot be taken during pregnancy and can cause severe birth defects in the baby.

Tips for Coping with Infertility

Of course, if you are a single woman or in a lesbian or gay relationship, you knew ahead of time that you need treatment and this may not have been such a big adjustment. But for a couple who had no idea they had such a severe fertility problem, the diagnosis can be devastating. It is really important to take the time that you need to grieve the fact that you need treatment to help you conceive. Dealing with your emotions can help you move forward in a positive manner, and be ready for treatment. Being resentful and denying the need for treatment is not a healthy way to move through treatment, nor is it healthy for your relationship with your partner.

ALERT

It's very important to work with your partner as a team when it comes to dealing with infertility. Have a discussion before you start treatment to figure out how much you can afford to spend, what your plan will be and at what point you will look for alternative methods to build your family.

Now is the perfect time to pick up a new hobby, take that dance class you've always wanted to, or pick up your paintbrush again. Even better, take that cooking class with your partner. It's a great way to spend time together outside of the doctor's office and gives you a chance to talk to each other about something other than sperm counts and estrogen levels.

Talking to Your Family

Making the decision to tell or not tell your family can be a tough call and is only complicated by family dynamics and politics. There is no right answer, only what is right for you or you and your partner. Do you even feel comfortable talking to them about such a touchy subject? Are you planning on telling your child about his unique origins? That decision alone can play a huge role in whether or not you tell the rest of your family.

When to Consider Telling

It can be really helpful to have a confidant you can trust and unburden your heart to. Infertility, and particularly the use of donated sperm (or eggs), is very stressful and can put a strain on your relationship. Having someone that you can cry and complain to, who isn't your partner, is a great way to get some of that stress out without blaming your partner.

Chances are that if you are in a lesbian relationship, your loved ones will figure it out that you got sperm from an outside source. However, don't feel the need to disclose the identity of your known sperm donor or that you used a sperm bank if you don't want to. A simple "that's private" or "we decided not to tell" should suffice in answering any questions that come up.

If you plan on telling your child when they get older, having your family support ahead of time can be helpful. That way there are no surprises when you do tell your child. It also gives them a chance to get used to the idea before your child finds out.

FACT

Whether or not you've decided to tell your family, it can be beneficial to have a group of supportive friends that you can talk to. Finding a support group, either in person or online, can be immensely helpful in working out some of the emotion surrounding infertility treatment.

When to Keep Quiet

Remember that ultimately this is a very personal decision between you and your partner. If you feel that your family will be rude or disrespectful toward you, your donor, or your child, it may be in everybody's best interests to keep this to yourselves, at least until they've had a chance to let the information sink in a little bit.

Your known sperm donor may also request that you keep the information to yourselves. He may have children who he doesn't want to find out just yet, or his family may not support his decision to have children outside of the family. Whatever the motivation, you should respect his wishes, as long as it's within reason. If disclosure to family and friends is an absolute must for you, and your potential donor doesn't share the same view, he may not be the right donor for you.

Disclosing Your Child's Unique Origins

Until recently, many families chose to not tell their children that they were the result of donor sperm. Current studies are showing that children who have found out as adults feel betrayed and resentful that such a huge secret was kept from them. Many even feel like they are missing out on a huge part of themselves and their personal history. The studies are finding that these offspring feel a sense of loss, that they are missing out on a chance to meet a whole other side of their family.

To Tell or Not

The official position by the ethics committee of the American Society for Reproductive Medicine, or ASRM, is that parents should disclose to their children that donated sperm or eggs were used in their conception. That being said, that decision is not right for every couple. Some families would not be accepting of a child conceived from donated sperm. If this is your situation, it may better for the child to not tell them until they were old enough to understand.

Keep in mind that children are incredible snoopers. They love looking through their parents' stuff and might come across some paperwork that would tell them about their conception. Children also ask lots of questions, and a well-meaning family may accidentally let the information slip. If you decide not to tell them, it might be a good idea to place all information related to their donor in a safe deposit box or other secure location where they will not be able to find it.

The Two-Week Wait

The two-week wait. What more can be said? This is the period of time right after you ovulated, when you either had sex, an insemination, or an embryo transfer, where you are waiting to see if the cycle worked. For many couples, this is the hardest part of the entire process. Nevermind the injections or the surgery or the daily visits—at this point, you're not doing anything but waiting.

There unfortunately isn't much that you can do to improve your chances of becoming pregnant at this stage. However, the best thing that you can do is really take care of yourself during this time. Relax, eat well, and get some sleep! Make plans to go out and see a show or something else to get your mind off the wait.

ALERT

Make sure to be diligent about taking your medication. There is a reason why the hormone supplements are prescribed, and messing with your dosage, or even skipping them altogether, can drastically affect your progesterone and estrogen levels, and potentially your pregnancy.

It's important to know that some women experience cramping and spotting during this two-week period. This can be the result of any number of factors, but it does not mean that you aren't pregnant. Sometimes when implantation occurs, women may notice a little cramping or spotting. The progesterone supplements themselves can cause both symptoms also. No matter what, do not stop taking your medication without talking to your clinical staff first, even if you are bleeding and swear that you are not pregnant. This bears repeating: Talk to your doctor/nurse before stopping any medication, no matter what is happening. They will best advise you what to do. Prematurely stopping your medication can cause you to lose the pregnancy, if in fact you are pregnant.

The Big Day—Your Pregnancy Test

Finally, the big day is here! Chances are, you're pretty nervous. Depending on what you tried that month, you may be asked to come into the office for a blood test, or you may be allowed to test at home using a urine pregnancy test. If you've done IVF or egg donation, you will most likely need to have the blood test. As part of your clinic's reporting requirements, SART will need to know how many patients were or weren't pregnant at the end of their cycle. A positive pregnancy test is a beta human chorionic gonadtropin level of above 5ng/ml.

That day, you'll likely be very nervous and anxious to get your results back. It can be helpful to think about where you'll be when you get the call. Will you be at work? Is that where you want to be when you find out you are or aren't pregnant? If not, make arrangements with the nursing staff beforehand. Maybe they can call your partner, who can give you the news later on. Or you can call at a designated time when you are on a break.

Unfortunately—and obviously—your pregnancy test can be negative. If that is the case, you'll stop taking your medication and wait for your period. You should also make an appointment to see your doctor in the interim. She'll go over all of the details of your cycle, including what she thinks went wrong and what your next steps will be. Sometimes, however, there is no clear reason why the cycle didn't work, and this can be incredibly frustrating. Rest assured, many couples fail a cycle, or two, or three, or four before they become pregnant. Failing a cycle does not mean that it will never work; it just means that that particular cycle didn't work.

If your test is positive, that's wonderful news! It can be such a relief to hear the good news after everything you've been through. You'll need to continue all of your estrogen and progesterone supplements (if you're taking them) until the doctor instructs you do stop, commonly around eight to ten weeks of pregnancy. Your reproductive endocrinologist will monitor your pregnancy in the initial stages, until you are ready to be discharged to your ob/gyn or pregnancy caregiver.

Depending on your medical history and the prognosis of the pregnancy, your doctor may recommend that you also consult with a specialist in maternal-fetal medicine. This doctor is specially trained to monitor women with high-risk pregnancies. The fact that your pregnancy was conceived through the use of IVF or using donated eggs/sperm does not mean that you'll need a high-risk specialist.

Pregnancy is a special miracle. Whether it was a natural conception or an assisted conception, it is still a miracle. There is nothing as exciting or life changing that you will ever experience. All of the planning and preparation you've put into getting healthy and staying healthy will help you ensure that your pregnancy and baby have a good start.

A "Premium Pregnancy"

If you conceived with the help of technology, you may find that people in the medical field view your pregnancy differently. They may look at your pregnancy as what is called a "premium pregnancy," a term that usually applies to a pregnancy where medical assistance was necessary. This can actually work to your detriment and may lead to unnecessary medical intervention. Discuss this phenomenon and use the information you get when deciding on a practitioner.

Remember that pregnancy is a natural state of being, no matter how you got that way. Your body does know how to be pregnant, so listen to the cues your body is sending you and respond accordingly. Use the team of care professionals you've assembled to help you look and feel positively toward your pregnancy. The power of positive thinking will take you far on the pregnancy and parenting pathway.

CHAPTER 20

Early Pregnancy

Congratulations! You're pregnant! After trying for so long and going through your infertility treatments, it's such a relief to finally hear the good news. The doctor still needs to make sure that your pregnancy is a good one, so you're not off the hook yet. Unfortunately, pregnancy loss and other complications are still a possibility. The doctor will monitor your pregnancy frequently in the beginning to watch for these complications.

bhCG Blood Testing

The beta subunit of human chorionic gonadotropin, abbreviated as bhCG, is the hormone that urine and blood pregnancy tests detect. Generally, lab values above 5ng/ml are considered positive. Some facilities may have different standards for what is considered a positive test, though. It is important to know, however, that just because a test is positive, it doesn't mean that the pregnancy will be good. For example, a bhCG level of 6.0 is considered to be a positive pregnancy test. But the level is so low that a good pregnancy is not likely.

Repeating the bhCG Testing

The doctor will likely ask you to repeat the testing every two to three days. This way the doctor can see how the bhCG level is moving. The number should double in two to three days to reassure the doctor that the pregnancy is progressing normally. If the level is not rising robustly, the prognosis for the pregnancy isn't great. Additionally, the bhCG testing can give the doctor an early indication of a possible ectopic pregnancy or even multiples.

Progesterone

The doctor will also likely check your progesterone level. Progesterone is the primary hormone of pregnancy, so it is important that you have enough in your body to support the pregnancy. If your progesterone level is a little low, the doctor may prescribe or change your progesterone supplementation to make sure that you have support.

FACT

Repeated progesterone in oil injections can be painful. Try applying an ice pack onto the muscle right before you take the injection. Afterwards, have your partner massage the area vigorously and apply a heating pad. The heat and massage can help break up the oil and make you more comfortable.

Progesterone supplementation can come in the form of intramuscular injections and vaginal suppositories. The doctor will choose the one that is more appropriate for you, based on your progesterone levels and medical diagnosis. You may even need to take both injections and suppositories to give you a sufficient progesterone level.

Ultrasonography

An ultrasound exam is a great way to learn a lot of information about your pregnancy. Early on in your pregnancy, ultrasound can see into the uterus to give you information like how far along you are, how many babies are in there, and where your pregnancy is located. This is an absolute sign of pregnancy.

Ultrasound can be used beginning around five to six weeks of gestation. The earlier it is used, the less you will see. At this point in your pregnancy, doctors will be looking for the gestational sac where your baby will grow. As the weeks progress, you will eventually be able to see your baby, and later hear the heart beat.

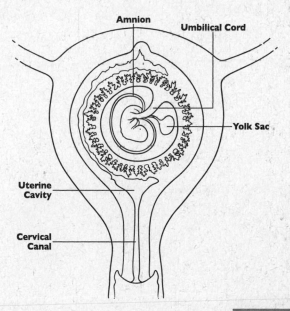

A six-week embryo

Ultrasound can be done abdominally. A wandlike transducer is coated in a special gel that helps transmit sound waves and is then run over your abdomen. For ultrasounds done very early in pregnancy, particularly weeks five through eight, an intravaginal probe is usually used because it allows the doctor to see in greater detail. This probe is covered in a plastic sheath, much like a condom, and placed inside the vagina right next to the cervix. This provides the best view of the contents of your uterus.

Abnormal Pregnancies

Unfortunately, pregnancies can be abnormal. From an early miscarriage to a life-threatening ectopic pregnancy, there is a lot of potential for some severe complications. Thankfully though, the serious ones are fairly rare. To make sure that your pregnancy is progressing normally, your doctor will ask you to have blood tests and ultrasounds somewhat frequently. While some minor cramping is normal in early pregnancy, make sure to report any pain or bleeding to your doctor so they can evaluate you if necessary.

Ectopic Pregnancy

Ectopic pregnancy is defined as a pregnancy that occurs in an abnormal place (in other words, the fertilized egg is implanted outside the uterus). More than 90 percent of all ectopic pregnancies occur in the Fallopian tube. Therefore, the more common name for this early pregnancy loss is called a "tubal pregnancy." Other locations of ectopic pregnancies can be the cervix, the ovary, the abdomen, or the cornua (the portion of the uterus where the Fallopian tubes enter) of the uterus.

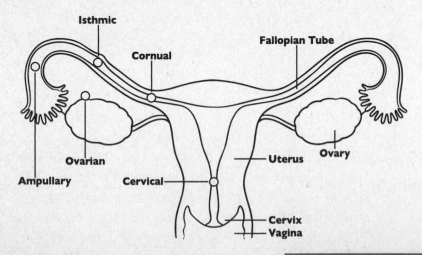

An ectopic pregnancy

This type of pregnancy is the leading cause of death for women in the first trimester. The warning signs can seem like other pregnancy losses, but include: bleeding from the vagina, abdominal pain or tenderness, shoulder pain, and/or weakness or dizziness. If you experience any of these, you should contact your doctor or midwife immediately to seek treatment.

Testing for ectopic pregnancy is difficult, because the answers are not always clear-cut, nor are they always available right away. Your hCG levels may be tested to check the rate of rise—they normally double about every two days in a normal pregnancy, but if the pregnancy is ectopic hCG levels may rise more slowly—though this alone is not an indicator of an ectopic pregnancy.

FACT

Even rarer is a heterotopic pregnancy, where one embryo implants in the uterus and another one implants in the Fallopian tube. The chance of a heterotopic pregnancy increases if you are going through infertility treatment, since you are having multiple embryos placed.

Ultrasound is frequently used, along with vaginal ultrasound, to try to visualize the pregnancy. If a uterine pregnancy is confirmed, then the chance of ectopic pregnancy is low. Sometimes it is too early to diagnose an ectopic via ultrasound, and the exam will have to be repeated later. If an ectopic pregnancy is visualized then you will proceed to treatment options available, depending upon your situation.

A laparoscopic procedure will be done in urgent situations to provide diagnosis and treatment. This is done in an operating room as surgery. Treatment for an ectopic pregnancy will always end the pregnancy. Unfortunately, there is no way to continue a pregnancy in these locations. Doctors do not yet have the technology to move the pregnancy to a viable location.

There are two main types of treatment for ectopic pregnancies: chemical and surgical. Chemical treatment is done with a drug called Methotrexate. It is used in nonurgent cases to dissolve the pregnancy without harming the tubes and other organs. Repeated hCG level tests will be taken to ensure that the pregnancy is dissolving and that further treatment is not needed.

Surgery is usually done in cases that are further along in their pregnancy or have another medical reason to not use the chemical process. It may be necessary, especially when the tube ruptures or there is other damage. Sometimes the woman will lose her tube and possibly her uterus if the bleeding can't be stopped.

Blighted Ovum

Blighted ovum is another form of early pregnancy loss. It is also known as an "anembryonic gestation." This means that a baby or embryo never forms.

Chromosomal disorders of the egg, or ova, are thought to be the main cause of this type of loss. It is usually detected during an ultrasound where a gestational sac is seen with no yolk sac or embryo. You may miscarry normally, the pregnancy may reabsorb itself, or surgery may be necessary to end this form of pregnancy.

Molar Pregnancy

Molar pregnancies occur when there is an abnormality with the placenta at the time of fertilization of the egg. They can be either "complete" or "partial."

A complete mole occurs when the nucleus of an egg is either lost or inactivated. The sperm then duplicates itself because the egg was lacking genetic information. Usually there is no fetus, no placenta, no fluid, and no amniotic membranes. The uterus is rather filled with the mole that resembles a bunch of grapes. The fluid-filled vesicles grow rapidly, which can make the uterus seem larger than it should be for gestational age. Because there is no placenta to receive the blood, typically you will see bleeding into the uterine cavity or vaginal bleeding.

ALERT

If you had a molar pregnancy, further pregnancy should be avoided for the period of one year. Any method of birth control, with the exception of an intrauterine device, is acceptable. This is to prevent further molar pregnancies.

A partial mole most frequently occurs when two sperm fertilize the same egg. There may be partial placentas, membranes, or even a fetus present in a partial mole. However, there are usually genetic problems with the baby, such as too many chromosomes. Rarely, a partial mole will exist with a twin pregnancy; however, the twin rarely survives.

Symptoms of a molar pregnancy can include increased nausea and vomiting, beyond normal morning sickness; vaginal bleeding; increased hCG levels; rapidly growing uterus for your pregnancy dates; pregnancy-induced hypertension prior to twenty-four weeks; no fetal movement or heart tone detected; and hyperthyroidism. Diagnosis is varied for this type of pregnancy loss. Most of the time a molar pregnancy will end spontaneously.

When the woman passes tissues that appear to be grapelike and shows them to her practitioner, then a molar pregnancy is suspected. Ultrasound can also help determine a molar pregnancy. When doing an ultrasound one sees a "snowstorm effect" on the screen. Serial hCG levels can show a rapid rise in hCG that may indicate that further study is needed.

There are a few treatments for a molar pregnancy. If the pregnancy has not ended on its own, a suction dilation and curettage (D&C) is usually used to evacuate the mole from the uterus. Induction of labor is not recommended due to increased risks of hemorrhage.

FACT

Once the mole has been removed, you will continue to need ongoing treatment. This includes testing hCG levels several times a week, then weekly, until they are "normal" for three weeks. Then you will be tested monthly for six months, and every two months until a total of one year has passed. A rising level of hCG and an enlarging uterus could indicate a choriocarcinoma, a rarer form of molar pregnancy, which is malignant.

Losing a pregnancy at any stage can be hard, and so there will have to be a healing time for all involved. You'll likely experience the stages of grief, though not necessarily in order or at the same time as your partner. What makes this type of loss different from a "normal miscarriage" or loss is the added concern of the mother's continued health, including the risk of cancer.

Miscarriage

Miscarriage is one of the most common forms of pregnancy loss. It has been estimated that up to 50 percent of all pregnancies will end in miscarriage, though many of these are pregnancies that the mother was not even aware of. Miscarriage is generally defined as the loss of a pregnancy prior to twenty weeks of gestation.

Many miscarriages occur very early in the pregnancy—sometimes so early that you may not have even known you were pregnant. Perhaps you thought your period was just a bit late or a bit heavy. This can be a sign of a very early miscarriage.

Types of Losses

There are several types of miscarriage. Spontaneous miscarriage, also called spontaneous abortion, means that your body completed the process and the uterus is empty. Incomplete or partial miscarriage could be a miscarriage in progress or one that has stopped prior to being completed. You may require a minor surgical procedure called D&C to help expel the rest of the uterine contents. There is also the threatened miscarriage, which is where you experience bleeding and/or cramping at any point early in pregnancy up to twenty to twenty-two weeks. Typically, since there is nothing that can be done to truly stop a miscarriage that is destined to be, you are told to watch for escalating signs of miscarriage (more bleeding, cramping, etc.). This crisis is over when you are either out of the danger zone date-wise or you cease having the symptoms.

A chemical pregnancy is a very early miscarriage; one takes place before the pregnancy can be seen on an ultrasound, usually before four to six weeks of pregnancy. You may take a urine pregnancy test, or have your blood drawn at the doctor's office and have the test come back positive, only to have it start to decrease a few days later. If your initial bhCG level is very low, it can sometimes indicate that you may have an early loss.

Bleeding in Pregnancy

Bleeding in pregnancy can be very scary. Here you've been wanting and waiting for this pregnancy and just when you think you've done everything...you're bleeding. The reasons for bleeding in pregnancy are many and varied. They can be caused by structural problems in the uterus such as a fibroid tumor. This might cause the sloughing off of some of the tissues in the uterus. This is particularly true if it grows or presses on the placenta.

ALERT

All bleeding in pregnancy should be taken seriously by you and your doctor or midwife. If you experience any bleeding or spotting, immediately call your practitioner. This means even if it's late at night or on the weekends. It is your practitioner's job to be there for you at all times.

Another potential problem with the placenta is called subchorionic bleeding. This is a small collection of blood just under the placenta. The blood seeps out from behind the placenta and enters the vagina. Then you notice the bleeding. This can be caused because of the area of implantation, or even trauma that the mother has experienced previously, such as a car accident or a fall.

Whether or not subchorionic bleeding will be problematic depends on the size and the severity of your bleeding. You will be tested by ultrasound, and the results will help your medical team determine your risk for complications in this pregnancy.

There are also times when you might experience bleeding and doctors can't find a cause or source. In these cases, you will be monitored closely. Remember to not panic if you experience bleeding. There may be a good explanation for the bleeding that is not immediately threatening to the pregnancy.

What to Expect in Early Pregnancy

When you think about pregnancy symptoms, a few probably come to mind right away, like morning sickness or a late period. These are both symptoms of pregnancy that you might experience, but not all symptoms of pregnancy are obvious. Some symptoms might be blamed on other causes at first—for instance, being tired might be blamed on the flu. Here are some symptoms of pregnancy that are fairly common and what you can do to survive them.

Morning Sickness

You might be pleased to know that only 75 percent of women experience nausea and/or vomiting with pregnancy. This symptom of pregnancy usually doesn't start until six or so weeks from your last period. You may experience just a slight queasy feeling whenever you get hungry. You might even feel your stomach churn with certain smells.

While it is called morning sickness, it can occur at anytime of the day or night. The morning period seems more common probably because women have empty stomachs and higher hormone levels. You can try eating a high protein snack before bed or even in the middle of the night to stave off the nausea. A handful of nuts or peanut butter crackers can work wonders.

Sometimes acupressure bands, worn like bracelets, can help you combat feelings of nausea and stop vomiting. These bands are used to put pressure on particular points on your wrists. They ease the feelings of nausea and in some instances reduce vomiting for you. You can buy them in many grocery, drug, or health food stores.

You will probably begin to feel this symptom ease around the end of your first trimester, or at about twelve weeks into your pregnancy. However, you might see a return of morning sickness later in pregnancy as your stomach space becomes more limited.

FACT

There is such a thing as too much of a good thing. While nausea and vomiting may reassure you that your hormone levels are up, you can vomit so much that you become ill, dehydrated, and malnourished. This is called hyperemesis gravidarum. Your practitioner can help you ease this symptom and maintain your health for your baby.

Fatigue

Not being able to keep your eyes open two hours into your day can be disheartening. but experiencing fatigue in your pregnancy is normal. Getting your work done or watching other children can be very difficult if you suffer from fatigue. To combat fatigue try to get a quick nap, exercise, and avoid caffeine, which will only send you up and then crashing down.

When you are feeling low about your lack of peppiness, remember that you are very busy growing a baby. Your body is rapidly changing, even if you can't see it. Your hormone levels are exploding, your uterus is expanding, and your blood volume is expanding as well. Give yourself a pat on the back and a break!

Sore Breasts

Ouch! Don't touch! You may experience breast tenderness during pregnancy. Or you may experience a heightened sensitivity—you may find that your sexual pleasure from your breasts is increased during this period of heightened sensitivity.

Breast tenderness is caused by pregnancy hormones, namely progesterone. Wearing a supportive bra can help with tenderness. Try wearing a sleep bra at night. This symptom usually diminishes during the second trimester.

FACT

While pregnancy symptoms can come and go, symptoms that completely disappear could indicate a problem. This is also true of symptoms that are severe. Never hesitate to call your doctor or midwife if you have concerns.

Frequent Urination

As your body changes and your uterus grows, you'll have more pressure on your bladder as well as more fluid to push through your bladder. This is a sign of pregnancy you can spot very early, and one that you will most likely experience. There is not much you can do about it.

Other Symptoms

There are plenty of other symptoms you might experience in early pregnancy. Two symptoms of pregnancy that many women experience are bloating or headaches. Some say that the taste of metal in their mouths was the first sign. Whatever it is you are feeling, be assured that someone else has felt that way before.

You might also be one of the lucky women who experience no symptoms of pregnancy. You could potentially glide through pregnancy with never a queasy feeling or a droopy eyelid. Congratulations if you are this lucky!

The best advice for dealing with pregnancy symptoms is to have a sense of humor and be prepared. If you find yourself feeling ill, keep a plastic bag and a towel nearby at all times. Keeping mouth rinse in the car isn't a bad idea either. If you're constantly hungry, carry snacks that are high in protein. Do what you can to minimize symptoms to make your life more comfortable.

Sharing the Good News

Finding out you are pregnant is a very exciting and nervous time in your life. Once you've had that positive pregnancy test, you are faced with many decisions, including when you should tell and whom you should tell.

Some people prefer to tell only their immediate family, choosing to wait until later in the pregnancy when the chance of miscarriage has dropped considerably before revealing the news to others. Others choose to tell anyone and everyone right away, reasoning that if they did have an early pregnancy loss, they would need the support of others.

FACT

Fear of pregnancy loss can prevent you from sharing your good news. If you've had a previous loss you can still go on to have a healthy pregnancy. Temper your fear with some excitement and consider telling very close friends for a support network.

Most people fall into a middle ground with whom they wish to share the news with. If you plan to keep your pregnancy a secret from some people in your life, make sure you know the integrity of the persons you are asking to share your secret. Nothing is more disappointing than calling someone to share your good news, only to find out that he or she already knows.

Reasons for not telling are varied, as mentioned before; early pregnancy loss is included in that list, as is the fear of reprisal from work, being judged differently by your peers, and personal acceptance. A lot of people decide to wait on revealing their joyous news until after the first trimester, when the miscarriage rates drop drastically. Others open up with the secret only as their abdomens begin to grow. If you have other children, you'll want to tell them the news before strangers can recognize your pregnancy by the size of your abdomen.

It can be difficult not to tell, for a variety of reasons. Severe nausea and vomiting may make it fairly obvious that something is going on, as will multiple visits to the care providers. If you are intent on not telling everyone, then you need to watch your actions. It's also hard not to scream with delight when you are in an emotional high.

There are a lot of creative ways to share the news of your new baby. Some people choose balloons with notes or frame ultrasound photos. Take a look at some of the more creative ideas at *http://pregnancy.about.com.*

The bottom line is to remember that you should tell people when you and your partner feel comfortable sharing your news. Have fun with it. Any way you tell people it is sure to be a moment that they will remember forever.

CHAPTER 21

Finding Support for Infertility

While undergoing infertility treatment, there is an abundance of information and places to get support. From formal counseling with a trained reproductive specialist to support groups online to pregnancy and infertility forums; there is a way out there for anybody who is trying to get pregnant. The trick is to find one, or several, that work for you. Finding someone who has been or is in your shoes is a great way to deal with a lot of the stresses and questions that often plague someone undergoing infertility treatment.

Reproductive Psychologists

Sometimes the need for support goes beyond what groups and meetings can provide. The issues that you find yourself dealing with may become too great to be dealt with in a peer support arena. You may be referred by your medical care provider or fertility specialist or even by yourself to someone who specializes in dealing with mental and emotional issues. While it may be hard to accept that you need this type of care, it is important that you seek help.

This person may be a psychiatrist or psychologist or other mental health professional. It should be someone who has the background and training to help you deal with the emotional issues that are surrounding your fertility. You may already know of someone, or you can look for someone through your health insurance.

FACT

Your fertility clinic may already have a therapist or counselor on board to help you if you decide you need his services. This person will have specific training and experience related to fertility issues. Do not hesitate to ask for a referral.

Sometimes the mental and emotional issues that come up are not really related to the issues of fertility, but simply to life in general. These stresses, combined with the stress of dealing with fertility treatments, may feel like too much to deal with. Seeking support by way of counseling can give you a one-on-one place to air your feelings without the fear of the information going anywhere else. It is a place to vent without worrying about what anyone else thinks or without worrying about who is listening.

You may even decide that couples counseling would be appropriate for you and your partner. Many couples find that this is a beneficial part of treatment for fertility issues. This is particularly true for dealing with guilt issues in a relationship.

Particularly stressful situations like that of a physical illness or situation like fertility treatments can create strains in any relationship. Treating them accordingly can help prevent the rift from becoming larger. It can also promote healing.

Infertility Organizations

There are a lot of organizations that have been formed to specifically provide information to couples that are suffering from all aspects of infertility. Many of these organizations can be found online or might even have local chapters that sponsor support groups and educational programs.

INCIID

The International Council on Infertility Information Dissemination, Inc., or INCIID (pronounced "inside"), is a very large organization that provides a wealth of information on infertility treatment. They also provide a scholarship and funding program to help couples finance their dreams of having a baby.

Besides infertility treatment, INCIID also provides information for couples who have made the decision to move beyond treatment and pursue alternative means for building their family. They can help you explore all aspects of both adoption and child-free living.

Resolve

Resolve is a very large organization that also provides a tremendous amount of support and education for couples suffering with infertility. They sponsor many webcasts and podcasts that feature experts talking about various parts of infertility, including finding an egg donor, pursuing adoption, and international surrogacy, just to name a few. In fact, if you have a question or are struggling with a particular area of your treatment, chances are they have a lecture from a well-known member of the infertility field about that topic.

In addition to education, they have a directory of support groups and ways to find support. Simply pull up the state you live in from a drop-down menu, and they will provide you with a list of groups, including contact information and more details about the type of group it is.

Fertile Hope/Livestrong

Fertile Hope is a part of Livestrong, the organization founded by cyclist Lance Armstrong. The sole purpose of Fertile Hope is to provide information to young men and women who are facing cancer and fertility-destroying treatments, about ways to preserve their fertility. Many young people who are diagnosed with cancer are never informed that they may lose their ability to have children as a result of their chemotherapy or radiation therapy.

FACT

Fertile Hope works with oncologists and other health care professionals to educate them on the preservation of fertility. They also work with fertility centers to arrange specially discounted programs so that people with cancer can afford the sudden expense of fertility preservation.

This organization seeks to reverse that. If your oncologist approves, you can sometimes go through a cycle or two of IVF in order to save the produced eggs for treatment later on. Of course, if your cancer is particularly aggressive or hormone sensitive, taking a few months off of treatment may not be an option. Men can easily bank sperm a few times for freezing. They also provide a great deal of financial information and support for adoption and egg/embryo cryopreservation.

Online Support

For a variety of reasons, infertility support groups are very popular on a web-based or Internet-based format. If you don't have a local support network, the web- or Internet-based groups can be a lifeline. This is one of the biggest benefits of online group support.

Some groups communicate in chat rooms, where you can talk back and forth in a real time environment while using a nickname. Chat rooms are relatively safe places to communicate, assuming you are not giving out your home address or other personal information. Most chat rooms allow you to talk about any subject you want at any point. It can be difficult to keep up with several conversations at once, but you will learn to either multitask or to focus on one conversation. Some chat rooms have a specific chat schedule and stick to it. Check with the administrators of the chat room for details.

Any information that you get via the web, Internet, or a support group should not be taken as personal medical advice. Always talk to your doctor about information you have learned online to see how it may affect your treatment.

You may also enjoy the Internet-based bulletin boards. This is a messaging system where you start discussions called threads. This is not done in real time, so you can browse topics and leave messages at will. It allows you to participate in more conversations at your own leisure. It is also done on a nickname basis.

You may decide that the online support groups provide a nice addition to your group meetings. By having a supplementation to the group support in between monthly meetings, you can feel a continuity of support. It also opens the base of people up that you are talking to and therefore it is more likely that you will find someone who has a history similar to yours.

Cycle buddies are a very popular thing on the Internet. A cycle buddy is another woman who is having similar treatments on or about the exact same day as your treatments. This allows you to commiserate with her and share a common experience.

While the Internet may be a great way to have support in an anonymous environment, there is some indication that if you seek support via the Internet, you are less likely to seek support in real life.

Regular users of Internet chat rooms may sound like they speak a different language the first time you see it. You will quickly learn the many different acronyms. Here is a quick list to help get you started.

▼ **INTERNET CHAT ROOM TALK**

Abbreviation	What It Means
2ww	Two-Week Wait (Waiting for your period)
AF	Aunt Flo (Your Period)
BBT	Basal Body Temperature
BCP	Birth Control Pills
BD	Baby Dance (Sexual Intercourse)
CD (cd)	Cycle Day (usually followed by a number)
CM	Cervical Mucous
DPO	Days Post Ovulation (usually followed by a number)
EWCM	Egg White Cervical Mucous
HPT	Home Pregnancy Test
HSG	Hysterosalpingogram
IUI	Intrauterine Insemination
IVF	In Vitro Fertilization
LMP	Last Menstrual Period
LP	Luteal Phase
M/C	Miscarriage
O or OV	Ovulation
PG	Pregnancy/Pregnant
SA	Semen Analysis

Finding support is always a great thing to do! Whether you find that support online or through a support group, it's highly recommended that you and your partner have outlets other than each other.

Your Marriage and Sexuality

During the process of being treated for infertility you will be physically poked and prodded in very personal ways. Your partner will also be poked and prodded. This process can really wear you down, leaving you with very little reserve left to help the other parts of your relationship.

Confronting Your Emotions

You or your partner may go through different emotions regarding your treatment. You may see highs and lows. You may experience depression, anger, guilt, and grief. These are all normal emotions to experience. The problem is that you are not necessarily experiencing them at the same time or in the same manner.

Communication with your partner is the key to helping your relationship survive the trials and tribulations of infertility treatments. Remember, the goal of treatment is to have a child together. Therefore, it is essential that you keep your relationship strong and steady so that you can be together in enjoying the child that will hopefully be a result of your treatment.

Some couples report that they have a lot of trouble communicating. Some express that their guilt over being the one with the diagnosed fertility problem weighs heavily on them. They feel like they are unable to give their partner the child that they desire. This leads to a variety of problems.

Whose Problem Is It?

Sit down and talk at length about how you feel with your partner. If you are the one with the fertility problem, be sure to let your partner know how you are feeling. He will be able to reassure you that you still have his love and support.

FACT

While your fertility treatments may bar you from having sex at certain times, there are other ways to physically express your love together. Try getting a book on sensual massage. Take a romantic walk or have a candlelit dinner to help rekindle some of the romance that you may feel is lacking from your life.

If you are not the one with the fertility problems, you can reassure your partner that you do not blame him for the problems. Remember that your goal is to have a child with your partner. Explain that you are willing to walk this road with him in order to have that child, no matter what it takes to bring that dream into reality.

Remember also to talk about your fertility issues outside of the bedroom, and leave your intimate moments reserved for talk of your love for each other, not fertility or fertility treatments.

Sometimes taking a break from fertility treatments is necessary to work on your relationship. It can be a good source of stress relief simply to not worry for a period of time about doctor's appointments and testing. Use this break to work on your relationship outside of family as well. Having a strong support group is essential no matter what path you ultimately choose to take.

Finding Help after Pregnancy loss

Anyone who has lost a pregnancy, at any stage, knows just how devastating it can be. For the couple that has undergone multiple IVF or infertility treatments, this is especially true. After investing so much, both emotionally and financially, it seems tremendously unfair to finally get your positive pregnancy test, only to suffer a miscarriage.

Emotions after Pregnancy Loss

Everyone deals with their grief in a different way, but there are several steps that everyone goes through in their journey through it. One well-known theory suggests that there are five stages of grief. The first stage is denial. You may not believe that you really lost the baby; it must be a mix-up in the lab, or something else. Next is anger, followed by bargaining, depression, and finally acceptance. Everybody will progress through the five stages at a different rate. Some people may move forward, and then regress as time goes on. Some people even skip certain stages.

Physically, you may feel fine. Some couples may have difficulty eating or sleeping, or they may eat and sleep more than normal. Some women cry; others don't. As you can see, your grief is completely your own. How you deal with it is your own, too.

Finding Ways to Heal

Finding a way to move through the grieving process and eventually healing is a must. Not properly dealing with your grief makes it more likely that you will suffer from a severe depression. Don't be afraid to ask for help if the loss becomes overwhelming; and don't ever worry that it's too early in the pregnancy for you to need to grieve. A woman can bond with her pregnancy as soon as she hears that she is pregnant, and that doesn't change if she is early or late in the pregnancy.

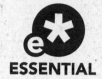

ESSENTIAL

Not dealing with your grief can quickly lead to depression. While it is important to move through the feelings that you have, people who suffer from dysfunctional grief patterns are not able to move on after a loss. Getting help is a vitally important part of recovering from a loss.

If your loss was late in the pregnancy, see if you can hold the baby or take her picture. Having a memorial service, even if it's just your immediate family, can be incredibly beneficial in helping you begin to acknowledge and move through your loss. Of course, this isn't possible with an early loss, but perhaps you have other mementos of the pregnancy that you can save; your sonogram results, the journal entries that you wrote when you found out that you were pregnant, or even your lab results. Some couples choose to put those items in a special place like a photo album or scrapbook. Others just tuck them away where they know they will be able to find them.

Living in a Fertile World

What do you do when your third baby shower invitation this month comes in the mail? You begin to dread the mail as much as you dread seeing your period. Not to mention, you may feel like your friendships are beginning to suffer because of your feelings.

The fact is there will always be someone having a baby. You will always run into pregnant women at the mall, even if you go out of your way to not pass any maternity or baby-related stores. The pregnant population will find you.

Coping Strategies

You need to develop good coping strategies for dealing with the feelings that arise from seeing pregnant women and babies in your life. Sometimes you may choose to avoid being in situations with pregnant women and babies. Other times you can't get out of the situation. By knowing ahead of time how you will deal with it, you can more easily accept the situation.

If the people in question are relatives or good friends, you may want to sit down and talk to them about how you are feeling. If they know about your struggles to conceive they themselves may be unsure of how to behave or act around you. Help them by spelling out for them what you need from them. You might tell a good friend that you'd love to come to her baby shower, but that it's too painful for you to be there. Explain to her how happy you are to be invited to celebrate and that you really are excited for her, but that you are simply too overwhelmed to attend.

If you find that your friends are *not* inviting you to baby showers or other baby-related functions, and you are equally offended by this, remember that most likely they are trying to spare your feelings. Be honest and tell people what you want and need. They are not mind readers and are probably making the mistake out of kindness.

In situations where you do not feel comfortable sharing your personal struggles, you may choose to simply invent an excuse to leave or walk away until the conversation turns to something else. Steer the conversation in another direction yourself. If you have a friend with you who does understand, look to her for support in making this change.

Hearing friends and acquaintances complain about pregnancy symptoms or losing those last few pounds of baby fat can really grate your nerves; you can either walk away or simply ask them to refrain from complaining around you.

The keys to dealing with issues of everyone else being fertile can be difficult and overwhelming. There will be times when it is possible for you to be around others who are obviously fertile. Tell those who are closest to you how they can help you and what you need from them. True friends will do their best to accommodate you. To those that you are around who are not privy to your fertility struggles, turn a deaf ear and move on whenever you politely can.

CHAPTER 22

When It Doesn't Work

For some couples, their journey toward parenthood ends without a pregnancy or the children they had been hoping for so desperately. While some couples do choose to not have children, there are other options for couples who want to expand their family. Becoming foster parents or adopting children, or even embryos, are all excellent alternatives if you and your partner are open to them.

Second Opinion

There may come a point where your doctor says that there isn't anything else she can do for you. She doesn't believe that further treatment will be beneficial or is likely to work. Or, there may come a point where you have tried several cycles and you no longer feel comfortable working with your doctor. It may be time to get a second opinion.

Many couples do this, and your doctor will not be insulted. It may be that another clinic has protocols that are better suited to your particular situation, or that the doctor has more experience in dealing with people with your diagnosis. Ultimately, your doctor wants you to get pregnant. If she is not able to do it, she will encourage you to find someone who can.

Couples often tend to get a second opinion before moving onto care using an egg donor or gestational carrier. That is a huge step for many people and they want to exhaust all other options before going down that road.

Getting a second opinion that confirms the first can help you come to grips with what you must do, be it use an egg donor or carrier, or even give up treatment. You should never feel forced into doing something that you are not ready for, and getting another expert's opinion can sometimes help you make the difficult decision.

Making the Decision to Give Up

Making the decision to give up is never an easy one. Perhaps you've exhausted your financial resources. Maybe it's your emotional reserves that have taken a beating and you're not sure you want to continue. Or it might even be your partner who's ready to throw in the towel and look for alternatives. Whatever the reason, it can be an extremely difficult decision to stop treatment and come to terms with the fact that you will not have a biological child.

When Should You Give Up?

There's no right answer for that one, as every couple will know what is right for them. Some couples don't want to go through, or have the means to go through, IVF. Others will do multiple cycles of IVF, but never with an egg or sperm donor. Still others will exhaust every means possible, including IVF, donated eggs and sperm, and even using a gestational carrier.

You should talk to your partner before you start treatment, so you both understand and come to a consensus as to what that threshold is for you as a couple. This eliminates the need to make important decisions when you are feeling particularly emotional.

FACT

If you and your partner are toying with the idea of giving up but aren't 100 percent sure, maybe a vacation or break is in order. It doesn't have to be an actual vacation—though that isn't a bad idea—but just some time off from treatment can be enough to gain some perspective into what is best for you and your partner.

If You and Your Partner Don't Agree

Quite often, one member of a couple reaches the decision to end treatment before the other and this is perfectly normal. So what are you to do if you are ready to stop, and your partner isn't, or the other way around? Start by talking to your partner about his motivations to stop or continue. Is he emotionally spent? Concerned about the finances? Remember to listen and communicate in a positive manner, as this conversation might be difficult. If there is a way to come to a compromise, try and work one out together. Maybe you agree just one more cycle, or that you'll look for alternative funding programs. If you absolutely cannot come to an agreement, speaking with your doctor or a marriage therapist may be in order.

Child-Free Living

There are many couples that decide to live their life without having children, and they often lead quite fulfilling lives. If you love being around children, there are lots of ways that you can enjoy a relationship with them without having any of your own. Having a special bond with your nieces and nephews is a great way, especially if you live close to them. You can also volunteer your time with Big Brother/Big Sister or other mentoring organizations where you are matched with a child who is in need of your time and attention.

Making the decision to live child-free is a big one, and not one to be taken lightly. There are definite advantages and disadvantages to child-less living. Many couples opt to travel quite a bit with their extra money and time. Becoming a volunteer or missionary with your church, the Peace Corps, or an international orphanage can also be quite fulfilling. Others dedicate their time to mastering a skill that they wouldn't have time for otherwise, like a sport or a language.

FACT

When you choose to live child-free, you will have lots of time to foster your personal relationships, and especially the relationship with your partner. You can go to (or skip!) a night out on a minute's notice without having to worry about a babysitter.

Of course, there are disadvantages as well. Sometimes families are not as understanding about your choice to not have children. This can cause discord and resentment and a whole lot of questions about your lifestyle. Quite often, couples are concerned about who will take care of them in their old age. They also want someone to pass down their traditions and family values to as they get older. But couples facing a child-free life should remember that they have lots of other family members and friends who can help them as they get older. There may also be nieces and nephews, or a friend's children who will be quite willing to pass those memories along.

Adoption

The adoption of an infant is absolutely nothing new; it is something that has gone on, officially and unofficially, since the beginning of time. Adopting a baby is still a great way to start a family today.

The process of adopting varies from state to state and country to country. Be sure to find out all of the requirements for your state before proceeding with the adoption process. The same is true if you are looking at adopting a child from another country—rules vary widely, so it's best to know what you're getting into.

Adoption means that you and your partner agree to legally become parents of a child that is being given up by her birth parent(s). The ages and abilities of children up for adoption will vary widely. You may be limited on whom you can adopt based on what you and your spouse can offer according to a home study (an analysis done by an adoption agency that determines your readiness to adopt).

FACT

Many families anticipate that adoption is the answer to their financial woes in terms of adding to their family. But adoption of any sort is likely to cost you a lot of money for the legal proceedings, home studies, and other expenses that are likely to come up.

You may or may not know the parent(s) of the child being placed for adoption. You may or may not ever have contact with them. Sometimes this decision is up to you. Sometimes this decision is totally up to the birth parent(s).

Getting Ready

You will have to open your lives to the courts and adoption services agencies. They will look at every part of your lives. A state-sponsored agency first performs a home study. Your lives and home are scrutinized closely to ensure that you are prepared and your home is suitable for bringing a child into. This can be a very stressful and unsettling time in your life. Even if you decide to adopt from another country, you will need to do a home study.

FACT

The rates of adoptions vary widely depending on region, ethnicity, age, and so on. The National Adoption Information Clearinghouse (NAIC) maintains statistics on adoption: *www.calib.com/naic/stats*.

Talk to other parents who have become a family through adoption. Join a support group. Talk about issues specific to adoption. The emotional ramifications are great, and you and your partner may not agree on many issues. Again, communication regarding these issues is very important. For some families, the lack of a genetic link to a child is something that they cannot get past. Make sure you are comfortable with this aspect, as this is a central point of adoption.

Find out what you need to know about adoption in your area. Talk to your spouse and your fertility center. You can get referrals for different types of adoption, including the adoption of older children, special needs children, and so on.

Agency Adoption

Most states have a state-run adoption agency or organization. This is probably the most well-known method of adoption. The benefits of using a government agency are that they have more experience and oversight of the process than many of the independent adoptions. They are very familiar with the procedural aspects of adoption. The downfall may be the length of the waiting list to adopt a baby, particularly healthy newborns.

Independent Adoption

If you find that the waiting lists in your area are long, you can try to get involved in independent adoptions. This is a bit more time consuming, but may be a faster way to adoption than other methods, though not always and not without cost. This means that you and your partner advertise that you are looking to adopt a baby. You will typically work with a lawyer or an adoption agency to help you find a birth mother, which is usually done prior to the birth of the baby.

Some agencies or lawyers will place ads looking for mothers who are interested in placing their babies for adoptions. Other groups work solely with agencies that run homes for teens or other unwed mothers. The agency or lawyer finds the mothers, and you are introduced to them by way of a letter and/or photo of your family, explaining why you wish to adopt a baby.

The truth is, healthy infants are hard to find for adoption. You may hit stumbling blocks in trying to adopt special-needs infants or children. You may run into the same difficulties in interracial adoption as well.

Adopting Out of the Country

Many people are choosing out of country adoption for a variety of reasons. In 1999, the National Adoption Information Clearinghouse (NAIC) estimated that U.S. citizens adopted 16,396 foreign-born children. But it's not necessarily faster, cheaper, or fraught with any less red tape.

Many couples are finding out that adoption from out of the country poses its own risks and problems. From visas to fears of disease, the emotional and financial strain of international adoption is great. This is not to say it is impossible, because these hurdles are true of most forms of adoption. But be prepared and know the process by talking to other families who have experienced the same thing.

Adoption can be a great option for building your family. While it does not involve the physical pain of fertility treatments, it is still a source of financial and emotional strain. The good news is that adoption from all sources is a great way to bring you together with a baby to help build your family.

Foster Care

Taking care of children who have been placed into foster care can be a wonderfully rewarding experience for the right people. After all, nobody needs the love and support that good parents could provide more than those foster kids. However, this is not the right choice for everybody.

Is Fostering a Child Right for Us?

Many of the children who are in foster care have seen the very worst that life has to offer. They have been the victims of abuse and neglect and may not have ever had someone they can trust and depend on. As a result, foster kids often have a lot of difficulty adjusting to their new lives and can act out significantly. You are also taking the risk that the child can be taken from home and placed back with their parents or other relatives, regardless of how much you've bonded with them. This can be heartbreaking, especially if you know that the child isn't being returned to a positive situation.

That being said, you know that you are having a tremendous impact on the children you foster. Sometimes foster parents can even adopt the child they are fostering, if that child has no other options for a permanent guardian.

How Do We Become Foster Parents?

There are lots of requirements that must be met before you and your partner can take in your first child. You must take a class to learn about how to deal with the unique challenges that come up when you foster a child. You and every member of your household will need to undergo a background check, criminal record check, and fingerprinting. Your home will be inspected to make sure that you have an adequate amount of room (and beds) to take on an additional child.

If you are thinking about fostering a child, you should check out *www .nfpainc.org/content/index.asp?page=FAQ&nmenu=3* for more information on the requirements and experiences of foster parents.

You will be interviewed to assess your emotional and family stability, and your willingness to work with the agency that places a child with you. While there is financial assistance provided by the state, they will want to ensure that you are making a sufficient income so that you are not dependent on the aid for survival. Finally, you may need to obtain character references and recommendations as well.

Embryo Adoption

You will probably not hear much talk about embryo adoption, most likely because there are a lot of potential problems with embryo adoption; however, it is done in many places.

What exactly is embryo adoption? Embryos from eggs that were fertilized and then either abandoned or given up for adoption are implanted in another woman. The legal issues involved here are amazing. In some states, couples are required to legally adopt a child conceived from an embryo that is not genetically linked to the mother, even if the mother carries the child in pregnancy and gives birth to that child.

You may decide that embryo adoption is a great option for you and your family. It gives you the ability to experience pregnancy and birth, even if you are physically unable to provide the egg or your partner cannot provide the sperm. You may prefer embryo adoption to live infant adoption so that you can control the prenatal variables, such as medical care and exposure to harmful substances. It may also be less expensive than traditional adoption.

Why would someone give up an embryo for adoption? They may feel that it is a morally good thing to do, rather than allow the frozen embryos to stay in the clinic or to be used for medical research. The couple for which the embryos were originally intended may now be unable to use them for medical or social reasons. Perhaps they have even completed their family and now wish to help other infertility patients complete their own family.

However you decide to expand your family, it's a very special time in your life. Adjusting to your new child can definitely provide some challenges, but it will also be a wondrous time in your life as you get to know this special person that you worked so hard to meet. Prepare yourself for a healthy pregnancy and delivery, or adoption if that's the road you choose. Best of luck to you and your family!

Your Infertility Treatment Organizer

Fill out this questionnaire and bring it with you to your first appointment. It can help you organize all of your thoughts, medical history, and the questions you want to ask the doctor, so you don't forget anything!

My medical history: _____
_____
_____

My surgical history: _____
_____
_____

My partner's medical/surgical history: _____
_____
_____

My first period: _____
My last period: _____
How long between periods? _____
Concerning symptoms: _____
_____
_____

My pregnancy history: _____
_____
_____

Pregnancy losses:
_____
_____

Questions to ask the doctor:
1. _____
2. _____
3. _____
4. _____
5. _____

Next steps: _____
_____
_____

APPENDIX B

Additional Resources

Fertility-Related Organizations

American Society for Reproductive Medicine (ASRM) (formerly the American Fertility Society)
1209 Montgomery Highway
Birmingham, AL 35216-2809
(205) 978-5000
www.asrm.org

ASRM provides patient and physician information. They also help govern and provide guidance for fertility programs both in training and in ethical situations. You will find great handouts on various positions from ASRM here; also available in Spanish.

Society for Assisted Reproductive Technology (SART)
1209 Montgomery Highway
Birmingham, AL 35216
(205) 978-5000 x109
www.sart.org

SART runs the statistical information processing that will help you compare fertility clinics. It is the place you'll find the most information, and should be consulted when trying to decide what program is right for you.

The International Council on Infertility Information Dissemination, Inc. (INCIID)
P.O. Box 6836
Arlington, VA 22206
(703) 379-9178
www.inciid.org

Great information for support purposes. They offer chats with professionals for the layperson on various forms of fertility questions.

RESOLVE: The National Infertility Association

1310 Broadway
Somerville, MA 02144
(888) 623-0744
www.resolve.org

Primarily an organization for persons interested in receiving support for various fertility issues. There are some great leadership positions filled in this organization by professionals in the field as well as parents.

National Adoption Information Clearinghouse (NAIC)

330 C Street SW
Washington, DC 20447
(703) 352-3488 or S(888) 251-0075
www.calib.com/naic

Information on adoption of any type in the United States and in foreign countries.

Organization of Parents Through Surrogacy (OPTS)

www.opts.com
Information to help connect people who have become parents via surrogates or who are interested in information on surrogacy.

Pregnancy-Related Organizations

American College of Obstetricians and Gynecologists (ACOG)

409 12th Street, SW
PO Box 96920
Washington, DC 20090-6920
www.acog.org

ACOG is the premier organization for obstetricians and gynecologists. They manage the postmedical school training and certification of this specialty. These physicians are trained in the care of the woman during all stages of life.

The Coalition for Improving Maternity Services (CIMS)
PO Box 2346
Ponte Vedra Beach, FL 32004
(888) 282-CIMS or S(904) 285-1613
www.motherfriendly.org

Established in 1996, the Coalition for Improving Maternity Services (CIMS) is a collaborative effort of numerous individuals and more than fifty organizations that represents more than 90,000 members. Their mission is to promote a wellness model of maternity care that will improve birth outcomes and substantially reduce costs. Here you will also find a lot of good information on choosing pregnancy practitioners.

Doulas of North America (DONA)
PO Box 626
Jasper, IN 47547
(888) 788-DONA
www.dona.org

DONA is the leading organization that certifies birth and postpartum doulas. A doula can assist the family before, during, or after childbirth. Using a doula has been shown to decrease the incidence of many complications of labor and postpartum, including Cesarean section and postpartum depression.

International Childbirth Education Association (ICEA)
PO Box 20048
Minneapolis, MN 55420
(952) 854-8660
www.icea.org

ICEA trains childbirth educators as well as prenatal fitness instructors throughout the world. Their website offers a search to help you find local instructors.

Lamaze International
2025 M Street, Suite 800
Washington, DC 20036-3309
(202) 367-1128
www.lamaze.org

Lamaze International is the leading certifying organization for childbirth educators. Promoting normal birth is the core of their philosophy as they train educators worldwide. Their site offers a directory, articles, and other interactive features.

Books on Fertility and Pregnancy

The Complete Guide to Fertility, ASRM, Ed.
Sandra Carson, MD, and Peter Casson, MD
This book was written and supported by members of the American Society for Reproductive Medicine (ASRM). It is a very technical book, but well worth the read.

The Everything® Pregnancy Fitness Book
Robin Elise Weiss, LCCE, ICCE-CPE, CD (DONA)
This book is a great overview of exercises for each trimester. The photos are clear and the text succinct. It includes special chapters on exercising in special situations like bed rest and includes a postpartum workout as well.

Getting Pregnant Naturally
Winifred Conkling
This book focuses on low-tech ways to help you get pregnant, including homeopathy, acupressure, nutrition, lifestyle changes, and more.

Overcoming Infertility: A Guide for Jewish Couples
Richard V. Grazi, MD
This book is a great resource for observant Jewish couples and the unique challenges they face when pursuing infertility treatment.

The Pregnancy Book

William Sears, MD, and Martha Sears, RN, IBCLC

This doctor/nurse, husband/wife team tells it like it is about pregnancy and birth. They lay it on the line about the choices you have and the healthiest approach to pregnancy. It is laid out in a convenient month-by-month format to help you find the information you need, when you need it.

Taking Charge of Your Fertility

Toni Weschler, MPH

This is an excellent manual for learning about charting your natural fertility cycles. It goes into very great detail about symptothermal testing and charting your basal body temperatures.

Websites

About Adoption Guide

Nancy Stanfield's guide to all types of adoption has you covered from the decision to the execution. She has a great website on dealing with the emotional and financial issues of adoption.

http://adoption.about.com

About Infertility Guide

Infertility from diagnosis to high-tech assistance. Includes a personal touch with lots of opportunities for loving support from others in your situation. A great place to look for cycle buddies.

http://infertility.about.com

About Pregnancy Guide

Pregnancy-related articles including a pregnancy calendar, ultrasound photos, community support, belly gallery, and other pregnancy-fitness related resources.

http://pregnancy.about.com

Childbirth.org

This pregnancy website is dedicated to helping you maintain a healthy pregnancy. There are many informative articles on all aspects of pregnancy, and fun programs including the boy or girl quiz and birth plan creator.

www.childbirth.org

The Maternity Center Association (MCA)

This website offers consumer sections, including access to the electronic version of the book *A Guide to Effective Care in Pregnancy and Childbirth*. It also contains many tools to help you the consumer you choose the right care. It also includes a section on the rights of the childbearing woman.

www.maternitywise.org

Fertility Plus

A great site for patient- and consumer-driven information, including many Frequently Asked Question (FAQ) files and downloads like a basal body temperature chart.

www.fertilityplus.org

Couple to Couple League—Natural Family Planning

The Couple to Couple League provides trainings, in various locations across the United States, about how to use your body's fertility signals to help you achieve pregnancy and diagnose your cycle variability. This can be used to help achieve or avoid pregnancy with great accuracy. Their website includes information on finding local classes.

www.ccli.org

SHARE

SHARE is an organization dedicated to helping you grieve the loss of your child, no matter when your child died. Through a monthly paper newsletter that is free for the first year, to conferences held all over the United States, SHARE has support at heart.

www.nationalshareoffice.com

Index

We Have
EVERYTHING®
on Anything!

With more than 19 million copies sold, the Everything® series has become one of America's favorite resources for solving problems, learning new skills, and organizing lives. Our brand is not only recognizable—it's also welcomed.

The series is a hand-in-hand partner for people who are ready to tackle new subjects—like you!

For more information on the Everything® series, please visit *www.adamsmedia.com*

The Everything® list spans a wide range of subjects, with more than 500 titles covering 25 different categories:

Business	History	Reference
Careers	Home Improvement	Religion
Children's Storybooks	Everything Kids	Self-Help
Computers	Languages	Sports & Fitness
Cooking	Music	Travel
Crafts and Hobbies	New Age	Wedding
Education/Schools	Parenting	Writing
Games and Puzzles	Personal Finance	
Health	Pets	